CW01335884

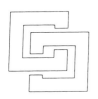

European Foundation
for the Improvement of
Living and Working Conditions

The Impact of New Technology on Workers and Patients in the Health Services

Physical and Psychological Stress

Loughlinstown House, Shankill, Co. Dublin, Ireland.
Tel: (01) 826888 Telex: 30726 EURF EI Fax: 826456

This publication is also available in the following languages:

FR - ISBN 92-825-6798-2
DE - ISBN 92-825-6799-0

Cataloguing data can be found at the end of this publication.

Luxembourg: Office for Official Publications of
the European Communities

ISBN: 92-825-6797-4
Catalogue number: SY-48-87-363-EN-C

Printed by the European Foundation

PREFACE

Since the end of the 1970s, the European Foundation has devoted several research projects to the relationship between new technology and physical and psychological stress.

The present report deals with the project which was started at the end of 1984, designed to investigate the impact of new technology on workers and patients in the health services.

Six reports presented, in their original languages, case studies carried out in member States of the Community (Denmark, Ireland, Italy, the Netherlands, the Federal Republic of Germany, and the United Kingdom).

The summary report, prepared by Dr Mike Fitter of the University of Sheffield, sums up the essential points made in these studies, and draws wider conclusions from them.

This research project is linked to two subjects of concern to the European Foundation: the question of working conditions for health service personnel on the one hand, and on the other hand the question of care and treatment conditions for the patients receiving this service.

The problem takes on major significance when one considers:

- that taking all levels and functions together the numbers of staff in this sector, according to the World Health Organisation, come to about three million people;

- that almost the entire population is in receipt of medical care under different guises (preventive treatment, curative treatment).

These two facts should also be seen against the background of rapid technological progress --- evidenced in spectacular fashion by certain surgical operations --- which is reshaping both the nature of treatment and the way in which it is provided, and in particular the relationship between users of the service and hospital staff. This progress is also accompanied by the democratisation of access to medical treatment, promoted especially by the decentralisation of treatment services and increased emphasis on preventive measures.

This is why the Foundation felt that a closer examination should be made of relations between technological change, work organisation, working conditions and quality of care, in an area which brings together all the developments already mentioned: the intensive care units within the hospital service.

In reading this study one should, however, beware of generalising the findings to all of these units, or even to the entire sector. The case studies carried out are in fact limited, both by their number and by their confinement to six countries.

On the other hand, these few cases serve to illustrate the kind of problems which are generally encountered. In this context, the evaluation process carried out with the social partners after the completion of the study confirmed the consistency of the findings here with those established in other settings. The cases also (and most importantly) serve to formulate recommendations concerning the management of change, especially where this bears on the introduction of new equipment and on work organisation.

The objective being pursued thus deliberately leaves out of account certain important points connected with technological development in the health sector, and especially the effects on the volume of employment.

Also left out of account is a question which would have necessitated a different approach, and even longer and more complex studies: 'the question of formulating recommendations not merely of a

methodological but also of a technical nature, concerning the design of monitoring systems used in intensive care services.

THE IMPACT OF NEW TECHNOLOGY ON WORKERS
AND PATIENTS IN THE HEALTH SERVICES:
(PHYSICAL AND PSYCHOLOGICAL STRESS)

(Consolidated Report)

By Mike Fitter

* * * *

University of Sheffield

June, 1986

LIST OF CONTENTS

ORIGINATORS OF THE CASE STUDIES

(1)   Mogens Agervold and Pia Ryom
University of Aarhus
Denmark

(2)   Eunice McCarthy
University College Dublin
Ireland

(3)   Sebastiano Bagnara and Paolo Legrenzi
CNR Rome   University of Trieste
Italy   Italy

(4)   Dylan Jones, Chris Miles and Alison Faulkner
University of Wales Institute of Science and Technology
UK

(5)   Adri de Vries, S H Schmidt, C van Ekeren and T F Meijman
Rijksuniversiteit Groningen
Netherlands

(6)   Ulrich Proll and Waldemar Streich
Gesellschaft fur Arbeitsschutz und Humanisierungforschung mbH
Dortmund
Federal Republic of Germany

SUMMARY

As part of its 1984/85 programme of work, the European Foundation for the Improvement of Living and Working Conditions undertook research into the impact of new technology on workers and patients in the health services. The terms of reference focused in particular on physical and psychological stress, as experienced by nurses and patients in a hospital environment. Reports from Denmark, Ireland, Italy, the United Kingdom, the Netherlands, and the Federal Republic of Germany have been submitted, and this report presents the consolidated findings from case studies carried out in the six European countries.

The research has theoretical foundations based on concepts derived from organisation theory and job design, and from stress research. The case studies aim to provide empirical evidence of the impact of new technology. However, the ultimate aim is to provide findings of practical relevance which may be used to improve the work experiences of hospital staff, and the service as experienced by patients. Within this framework the report makes recommendations on the way new technology should be developed and implemented within the health services.

The study focuses on the use of micro-electronic based technologies in hospitals. It is about the longer term impact of the technology, as well as the process of installing it and providing the necessary training in its use. The sources of stress in nursing work are of particular concern, as is the potential of new technology for alleviating or increasing job stress.

Intensive Care Units, including for example coronary care and neonatal care, have been identified as places which make substantial use of new technology, and are thus the focus for most of the case studies. Here the technology is used directly by nurses in the care of patients, and it is thus likely to have a substantial impact on nurses, patients and relationship between them. However, also of importance is the wider impact of new technology in the management of hospitals, and on the nursing process in particular.

Job characteristics and environmental stressors

A number of characteristics of nursing work emerge as commonly occurring stressors for nursing staff. These are:

(1)   A high work pace and frequent overload.

(2)   Rapid decision making and a high level of responsibility.

(3)   Cumulative work pressure, combined with shiftwork, that results in fatigue.

(4)   The difficulties of relating to seriously ill or dying patients and their relatives.

(5)   Working with inexperienced staff who cannot assume equal responsibility.

The following factors have been identified as relating directly to the use of new technology:

(1)   Enhanced cognitive demands required by complex equipment.

(2)   Poor design standards and equipment failures resulting in high levels of false alarms.

(3)   Lack of adequate training for nursing staff in the use of technology.

(4)   Ethical dilemmas concerning the use and non use of life maintaining technologies.

There is a problem of high workload, reported in all the case studies. It serves to magnify the effects of many of the other stress factors. There are a number of causes for this common finding:

(1)   There appears to be a general shortage of nursing staff in hospital units. This can be worse in low technology units because, in a situation of fixed overall health budgets, increases in resources for high technology units have the effect of 'draining' resources from other units.

(2)   Advances in medicine and technology make possible more diagnostic and therapeutic procedures. These involved the nurses in extra work.

(3)   The policy of reducing the time that patients spend in hospital intensifies the nurses' work.

Stress and coping

The case studies that have assessed stress levels experienced by intensive care nurses indicate that they do not report serious stress symptoms. Those that did show some symptoms tended to be the younger, relatively inexperienced nurses, with no prior work experience with new technology. Thus the extensive environmental stressors result in relatively mild stress symptoms. The nurses who reported most stress tended to resort to individual coping strategies. If nurses work in a supportive environment, and have the ability and opportunity to influence the sources of stress, they are less likely to experience stress. However, the time pressures created by a high workload provide little opportunity to participate in planning and other decisions which might make it possible to influence the work environment.

Using new technology

The majority of nurses see the benefits of using new technology, and in particular its life sustaining potential. However, they also experience serious problems with its use which stem from problems with design and reliability, and problems resulting from inadequate training.

The studies provided evidence that some nurses perceive an increased distance between themselves and their patients as a result of using the technologies. There is some variation in the extent to which nurses compensate for this distancing effect. In some environments there is little opportunity, in others the nurses provide additional direct support to alleviate some of the anxiety induced by invasive treatments.

Patients' responses to new technology

Generally patients have very positive views of the service they have received, and are particularly grateful to the nurses. They do not appear to experience any distancing from the nurses as a result of the technology. However, several studies reported that the technology and the physical environment can be intrusive and invoke anxiety. Invasive procedures also reduce patient mobility and bring greater risk of infection. The environment appears particularly stressful when patients are in a large ward with constant lighting and the distress of observing the suffering of other patients. In these circumstances patients may cognitively 'switch off', and exhibit symptoms of temporal-spatial disorientation, followed by almost total amnesia of their period in the ward. This has been referred to as 'Intensive Care Syndrome'.

Individual rooms may provide a more positive environment, adaptable to the needs of the individual patients. However, there may be negative consequences for the nurses who derive support from being with their colleagues and simultaneously being able to observe patients from a central point. Remote computer-based monitoring allows the nurses to monitor patients in single rooms from a central point, but makes direct observation difficult. However it may contribute to positive team work within the unit.

'Caring' and 'curing' aspects of nursing

'Caring' is the traditional autonomous nursing role to complement the 'curing' work of doctors. In modern hospitals it includes the basic physical care and psychosocial care that all patients need. 'Curing' on the other hand emphasises technical procedures, usually carried out for diagnostic or treatment purposes. Most curing activities are under the responsibility of doctors. The boundary between what doctors do and what nurses do is not well defined. It varies from unit to unit and, to some extent, depends on the availability of doctors, especially in acute situations.

The study poses the question, has the balance between caring and curing changed as a result of using new technology? The evidence indicates that many more curing activities take place in high technology units than in low technology ones. Correspondingly, low technology nurses carry out more caring activities. This appears to be a direct consequence of the vastly increased number of technical procedures entailed in the use of equipment in intensive care. It is also a consequence of patients spending less time in the hospital. In both types of unit nurses would prefer to spend more time on psychosocial care. The study identifies a 'hierarchy' of activities carried out by nurses:

(1)   Technical nursing.
(2)   Basic physical care and domestic duties.

(3)   Psychosocial care.

(4)   Organisational activities.

The general conclusion arising from the case studies is that caring and organising activities get squeezed due to the priority of technical procedures, combined with a shortage of available time. The extent of this squeezing seems to depend mainly on how much work pressure the nurses are under.

Recommendations

Summarised below is a list of seven recommendations, derived from the results of the case studies, and supported by the researchers who carried out the studies.

(1)   More or better training is required. This should be the responsibility of the hospital and not left solely to the equipment suppliers. It should include advice and support on how to integrate the technology into nurses' daily work, as well as providing instruction in functional aspects of equipment design and use.

(2)   The technology should be user-centred. Data collection should not interfere with the nursing process, but should support it. Nurses should be 'information users' and not just 'information providers'.

(3)   New technology increases the need for nursing support. A non-bureaucratic, supportive environment can reduce stress for nurses. Consideration should be given to whether there are adequate opportunities for nurses to communicate with each other, including when handing over to the next shift.

(4)   Care of patients needs to be ensured. The environment should be designed to allow normal sleeping and waking patterns wherever possible, and patients should have sufficient privacy. Since new technology is leading to relatively more curing activities, there should be a conscious and deliberate increase in the time available for caring activities.

(5)   Tasks, jobs and units need to be integrated. The development and
use of new technology is leading to increased specialisation in
nursing work. At the level of the tasks (curing and caring), the
job (technical nursing, domestic duties, social work, administration), and the unit (high technology, low technology) there is a
need for re-integration.

(6)   Nurses require more active participation in decision making.
Mechanisms should be set up to allow and ensure more involvement in
ward organisation, planning and policy making. In particular,
nursing staff should be actively involved in systems development and
implementation.

(7)   Increased staffing levels are needed. Work overload is the most
commonly reported stressor in nursing work. The most direct
improvement in patient care and the quality of nursing work would be
made if staffing levels were increased. This could enable the
implementation of the other recommendations.

1.0   INTRODUCTION

As part of its 1984/85 programme of work, the European Foundation for the
Improvement of Living and Working Conditions undertook research into the
impact of new technology on workers and patients in the health services.
The terms of reference focused in particular on physical and psychological
stress, as experienced by nurses and patients in a hospital environment.
Reports from Denmark, Ireland, Italy, the United Kingdom, the Netherlands,
and the Federal Republic of Germany have been submitted, and this report
presents the consolidated findings from case studies carried out in the six
European countries.

1.1   Aims of the Research

The first requirement in researching the impact of new technology in the
health services is to define and thus limit the concept 'New Technology'
and the settings in which it is used. In this study the term is used to
mean micro-electronics based technologies in use in hospitals. It is
likely that the technology will have been installed fairly recently, though
this is not a defining characteristic. The study is about the longer term
impact of the technology, as well as the process of installing it and
providing the necessary training in its use.

Intensive Care Units, including for example coronary care and neonatal
care, have been identified as places which make substantial use of new
technology, and are thus the focus for most of the case studies. Here the
technology is used directly by nurses in the care of patients, and it is
thus likely to have a substantial impact on nurses, patients and the
relationship between them. However, also of importance is the wider impact
of new technology in the management of hospitals, and on the nursing
process in particular.

The second requirement is to provide a conceptual framework in which the
impact of new technology can be assessed, and if possible improved. The
framework is developed in greater detail later in this chapter. The impact
can be direct, in that nurses and patients come into direct contact with
the technology. Thus it is important to determine personal experiences, to
ascertain attitudes, hopes, expectations, and anxieties about the
technology; and to assess its use by nursing staff. The impact can also

be indirect, for example, the impact on patients may be mediated by the work of the nurses and may be experienced through changes in patients' relationships with the nursing staff. The impact on the nurses can itself be a result of changes in work organisation brought about by the rationalisation of work processes resulting from technological change.

Thus a third requirement is to examine nurses' job content and the organisation of their work, and identify factors which generate stress (stressors) in their work. It is also important to identify job factors which do, or can, relieve or ameliorate stress and improve the quality of work for nursing staff. Within this framework new technology can be seen as an additional factor which may have a substantial effect on the work of nurses and their experience of stress. It is this area that has in the past received relatively little attention and is thus the focus of this study. For example, although it is generally accepted that technology can contribute to the 'curing' of patients, what impact does it have on the 'caring' provided by nursing staff, and on the inter-relation between 'curing' and 'caring' activities?

The research has theoretical foundations based on concepts derived from organisation theory and job design, and from stress research. The case studies aim to provide empirical evidence of the impact of new technology. However, the ultimate aim is to provide findings of practical relevance which may be used to improve the work experiences of hospital staff, and the service as experienced by patients. Within this framework the report makes recommendations on the way new technology should be developed and implemented within the health services.

1.2   Health Care and Nursing

A fundamental question which underlies all the activities of medical personnel, concerns the type of service they provide for ill persons (i.e. patients). This may have the purpose of returning patients to full health, or of preventing further deterioration. Traditionally the patient has been seen as an 'object', part of which is in need of treatment. This activity, which has been characterised as 'CURING' refers to the application of a medical technique which has been acquired during training. It focuses attention on the ill organ, the disorder, or the illness, and tends to relegate the patient to a passive role in the curative process. Curing is also seen primarily as being in the domain of doctors who may draw upon nursing staff to assist in the activities. It has been referred to as the 'medical model' of ill health. In the nineteenth century women were discouraged from practising medicine, since nursing was seen as their true vocation. This was made quite clear in a speech to the UK Parliament in 1875:

"God sent women to be ministering angels, to smooth the pillow, minister the palliative, whisper words of comfort to the tossing patient ill with fever. Let that continue to be women's work! Leave the physician's function, the scientific lore, the iron wrist and iron will to men!"

(Quoted in Faulkner and Arnold, 1985, p. 101).

Thus traditionally, nurses have been seen as providing a 'CARING' role, involving activities which provide for the basic needs of patients, and emphasise the psycho-social aspects of care. In caring activities patients are seen as individuals in interaction with their social environment, and from this perspective, rather than focus on the 'sick component', the patient is related to as a whole person.

The historical division of labour between male doctors involved in 'curing' activities, and female nurses involved in 'caring' activities still substantially exists, although boundaries and gender divisions are slowly changing.

Today, nurses carry out many activities, some of which are part of the patient's treatment and can be regarded as predominantly 'curing', for example changing infusion bottles, giving medication. Others can be still regarded as predominently 'caring' activities, for example meeting basic needs such as washing a patient, or psychological needs such as reassuring a patient or providing information on the situation at home. It is not necessary, nor is it frequently possible to classify activities as curing or caring, they will usually have elements of both, though with more emphasis on the one or the other. Some activities may indeed be neither, for example clerical procedures and other administrative activities undertaken by nursing staff. The main classification of nursing activities into four principal components is illustrated in figure 1.

A question which is of concern in this study is whether the <u>balance</u> of activities between the caring and other roles is changing for nurses. Historically the professionalisation of nursing has legitimated a range of activities by prescribing standards and educational objectives that qualified nurses must satisfy. The main areas of work undertaken by nurses in their care of patients are outlined below:

(1)   General physical and psychological care of patients.

(2)   Care, observation and treatment of patients in the light of their illness.

(3)   Counselling of patients and their relatives.

(4)   Communication with other members of staff, in and outside of the ward.

(5)   Recording information on patients and nursing activities.

(6)   Planning and managing their own work and that of subordinate staff.

(7)   Undertaking advanced training and instructing trainees.

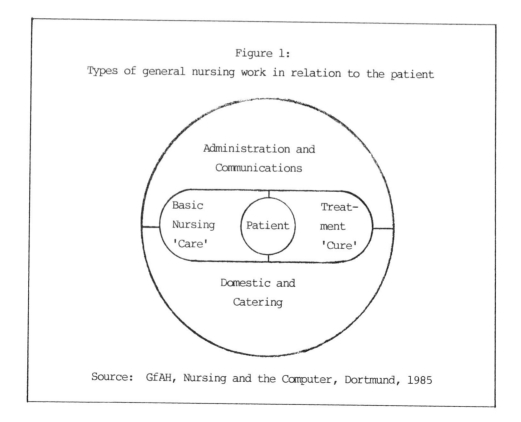

Figure 1:

Types of general nursing work in relation to the patient

Source: GfAH, Nursing and the Computer, Dortmund, 1985

Basic care is the central area of autonomous nursing, in which nurses' own professional skills and responsibility can be exercised. However there has been an increased emphasis on the curing role, and at the same time other specialist groups, for example psychologists or patient associations, have taken responsibility for some specific caring activities. Nurses' involvement in domestic and catering activities, for example bedmaking, meal distribution etc, varies from hospital to hospital, though there is also a tendency to make increased use of centrally provided services leading to more specialist domestic roles and removing many of these tasks from the nursing domain. New technology has led to the introduction of new activities which emphasise the curing role (i.e. focusing on the sick component rather than the whole person). This has resulted in nurses becoming involved in activities traditionally part of the doctors' treatment domain (Hannich et al., 1983), for example regulating the supply of medication, and has created role conflict, and potential stress, between the two professional groups. Technological change has also tended to increase the need for clerical work, and communications outside of the ward, for example requesting scientific tests and recording their results.

Thus an important question addressed in this study is whether the increased use of new technology has led to an emphasis on curing and administrative procedures at the expense of caring activities, or whether the technology has freed nurses time so that they can devote more time to their caring role. The Netherlands study in particular looks at this question in some detail and provides a quantification of the caring and curing components of nursing work in high and low technology units.

One factor which has contributed to a change in the balance of nursing activities is a widespread reduction in the period of time that patients spend in hospital. For example in the Federal Republic of Germany the average length of hospitalisation has dropped from 20 days in 1965 to 14.9 days in 1980. In the Netherlands it has dropped from 14 days in 1978 to 12.4 days in 1983. This change has not affected the amount of time spent on administration, diagnosis, and treatment related activities which tend to be concentrated at the beginning of the nursing process. The foreshortening of the patients' hospitalisation does however reduce the time spent on basic care activities which tend to be spread evenly across the period. Thus the net effect is to increase the proportion of nursing time required for administrative procedures and treatment. The shorter stay also means that patients are likely to require more attention from nursing staff while in the hospital.

The rapidly increasing costs of secondary (hospital) health care has placed greater strains on hospital resources. This has constrained, and in some instances reduced, the number of nursing staff available. The consequence of these factors is greater pressure on nursing staff and a feeling of being 'overworked'. It is against this background that the impact of new technology is being assessed.

1.3   Stressors in Nursing

A number of studies have been carried out in the past on stress in nursing work generally (Dohrenwend and Dohrenwend, 1974; Eden, 1982; Gray-Toft and Anderson, 1981; Jokinen and Poyhonen, 1980; Tabor, 1982; Vredenberg and Trinkous, 1983). The results point repeatedly to certain factors which must be considered as highly relevant and typical causes of stress. These factors are briefly described, with a view to identifying whether they lie in working conditions which could be affected and changed by the introduction of new technology.

(1)   Nurses feel a high level of responsibility for the well-being of patients who are sick, and perhaps dying. They must also deal with the emotional aspects of relating to patients and their relatives, frequently under considerable time pressure.

(2)   Generally nurses have a high workload with exceptional peaks, when for example new admissions occur. These events can create acute overload and possible stress reactions.

(3)   The work can be physically arduous involving lifting of patients and other heavy objects.

(4)   Shiftwork is the norm, and this is made more arduous by frequent overtime and the need to substitute for absent colleagues at short notice.

(5)   Conflict can occur with other professional groups, and with doctors in particular. Because doctors have authority for medical decisions nurses may have to seek permission for their actions, e.g. whether they can give a piece of medical information to an anxious patient.

(6)   Nurses can have responsibility for instructing trainees and super-
        vising junior staff. This can create stress, particularly when a
        shift is short of trained staff and is dependent substantially on
        inexperienced trainees.

(7)   The unpredictability of the work and of the patient's condition can
        create uncertainty as to the appropriate course of action or treat-
        ment.   If doctors are not immediately available this can be
        particularly stressful.

(8)   Medical knowledge and technology changes fairly rapidly, and thus
        nurses need regular training to keep up to date. Research has shown
        training often to be inadequate in the circumstances and this can be
        a source of stress.

Many of these factors are more stressful as a consequence of the increased
through-put of patients resulting from the policy of reducing the time that
patients spend in hospital.

The main factor which has been found to compensate nurses for this lengthy
list of stressors in their working lives is that the job is usually
regarded as highly meaningful, and valued by patients and society
generally. The work has many of the qualities regarded as good job
characteristics viz responsibility, meaningfulness, skill, variety, etc.
Also important for dealing with stressful situations is support from
colleagues and from superiors. Whether this is available will depend on
structural characteristics of the organisation (Gray-Toft and Anderson,
1981). In a positive climate nurses will perceive it to be possible to
influence events and avoid or minimise the impact of some of the stressors.
The evidence suggests that for the individual this is a better way of
dealing with a stressful environment than by individual 'coping' responses.

Some research has studied intensive care nursing specifically (for example
Bishop 1983; Claus, Bailey and Selye, 1980; Farmer, 1977, 1978; Huckaby
and Jagla, 1979; Jacobsen, 1978; Reichle,1975). The general finding is
that the above stressors also apply in intensive care but some are
experienced more intensely. For example patients are more likely to die,
and the work can be particularly demanding, physically and mentally. The
following account gives a vivid description of the nursing experience in
Intensive Care Units,

"The confrontation with suffering and death: probably the greatest and most agonising stresses are the inner mental conflicts. The subject is almost, or even completely, unaware of them and they are experienced as moods of diffuse depression or aggressive tensions, with feelings of hopelessness, resignation or irritation. From the constant confrontation with critically ill patients and their suffering, the hectic procedures of resuscitation, the feelings of inadequacy and guilt on the death of a patient, the pain of separation on the removal of a patient who has confided in one or with whom a compassionate relationship has been formed - all such continual confrontations, such constant psychological exposure to the risk of death, the agony of therapeutically necessary procedures, the pain of separation when the patient is transferred or dies - bring out all the apprehensions of life and painful memories which are repressed in everyone and are comparable to the shock of seeing a child who has been run over."

(Bernhard, 1983, p. 82).

Additional stress factors specific to intensive care are:

(1)   The ward environment is usually unrelentant. Bright lights are commonly on for 24 hours a day and are accompanied by regular noise of the equipment in operation.

(2)   Working with the technology creates additional pressures and requires additional knowledge and skills not part of a nurse's vocational training.

(3)   There can be a need for rapid and complex decision making if a crisis develops through a patient's sudden deterioration or by an equipment failure.

(4)   There is a substantial risk of accidents in intensive care.

(5)   When patients begin to recover they are usually removed to a less intensive ward, thus cutting off the potential for a nurse to relate to the patient at the point when it would be more easily possible.

However, Bishop (1983) has observed that "the emotional consequences experienced by nurses working in these units are barely mentioned" (p. 181).

Although the evidence shows that these additional stressors exist in intensive care environments they are to some extent compensated for because the positive aspects of the work are also experienced more intensely. That is the job is regarded as especially prestigious and meaningful.

1.4 Stress - Individual Responses to Stressors

Stress research has a long history, the current framework deriving from the work of Selye in the 1950s which was developed from a physiological-medical standpoint. He regarded stress as the non-specific response of the body to any demand made upon it (Selye, 1976). Thus although the environmental demands made on the body might be specific (the stressors) the response was non-specific, and could be construed either positively as 'energising', or negatively as 'distressing'. The body's response to negative stress is seen as having three phases:

(i)   a physiological <u>alarm</u> reaction, characterised by increased heart-rate, temperature and blood pressure

(ii) a physiological <u>recovery</u> in an attempt to adapt to the new situation, i.e. the physiological measurements return to normal

(iii) the control exercised in the second phase uses up physical and mental energies, thus if the source of stress continues the result is <u>exhaustion.</u>

The result of continuing environmental stressors can be 'burn-out syndrome' (Gray-Toft and Anderson, 1981). This is seen as a result of a high level of demands without the possibility of changing the underlying conditions, and the consequences in psychological and psychosomatic stress symptoms for the individual, followed by exhaustion, depression, alienation and apathy.

Workers have differing abilities to cope with a stressful environment and this has led some researchers to examine individual differences and 'personality factors' which might explain the differing responses to a similar environment. One important factor is the degree to which individuals perceive they have some control over their environment. Their real opportunity to control the environment depends, of course, on how amenable the environment is to change, and the <u>ability</u> of the individual to change it. For example, a nurse might successfully request a transfer to another ward. In a situation where it is not possible to change the source of stress, stress experienced by individuals will depend on their ability to adapt themselves, by changing their attitude, by 'turning-off' from the situation, or by temporarily removing themselves from the stressful situation and 'unwinding'. For example, facing problems with colleagues a nurse may focus all his/her energies on his/her own work and avoid distraction. However in a situation when patients die in the nurse's presence the only available stress reducing response may be to assume a detached attitude to patients and their families, and thus avoid becoming involved in their situation. From this view, stress is seen as resulting from any event in which environmental or internal demands (or both) tax or exceed the adaptive resources of an individual (Lazarus et al., 1980). Individual differences which are important include:

(i)   the extent to which a person's skills and abilities match the demands of the job, and

(ii) the extent to which the person's needs are met by the job environment (Caplan et al., 1975).

The factors which generate stress, and the characteristics of individuals which influence their response to it, and thus determine their 'stress reaction', are outlined in figure 2. This figure represents the framework in which the case studies can be assessed later in this report.

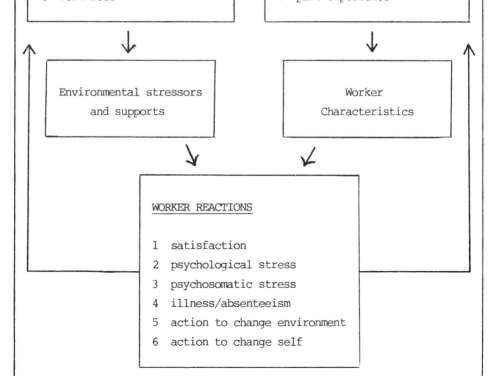

Figure 2:
The stress model with its environmental and worker variables

WORK ENVIRONMENT (physical and psychosocial)

Technological
1 physical/chemical factors
2 'new technology'
Organisational
1 quality of work
2 co-operation/conflict
3 controlability/discretion
4 work role

THE WORKER (physical and psychological resources)

1 age, sex etc
2 physical characteristics
3 qualifications/skills
4 learning potential
5 needs and expectations
6 personality characteristics
   e.g. trait anxiety
7 past experience

Environmental stressors and supports

Worker Characteristics

WORKER REACTIONS

1 satisfaction
2 psychological stress
3 psychosomatic stress
4 illness/absenteeism
5 action to change environment
6 action to change self

1.5   New Technology in Hospitals

Medical technology has a long history of use in hospitals. Some of the earliest technology was concerned directly with patient monitoring and treatment, and it is out of this that the advanced systems to be found in Intensive Care Units have been developed.

Intensive patient monitoring involves some of the most sophisticated equipment currently in use by nurses. A typical feature of these systems is that patients are monitored continuously with the aid of technology attached with electrodes. Data on the patient's heart rate etc. is monitored and analysed so that warning signals can be given if irregularities occur. The data and analyses are usually available at the patient's bedside, and in some installations are also monitored in a central 'control room'.

The technology is therefore constantly vigilant of the patient's condition and alerts the nursing staff when necessary. This should offer a feeling of security to patients that they are being 'looked after', but may also create feelings of anxiety and alienation in relation to the 'technological' and strange environment, to having electrodes attached, the TV screens, alarms etc.

In addition to traditional nursing, the nurses' work consists of monitoring the equipment and responding to alarms. This requires new skills in order to be able to interpret and use the information coming from the monitoring equipment.

The increased use of technology has generally required more specialised skills and this has been a contributory factor in the reorganisation of hospitals into specialised health care units. Much of the advanced monitoring and treatment technology is now found in such units, which have also led to increased specialisation within the medical and nursing professions. Specialist units have also been created for carrying out clinical test procedures, for dispensing medication, and for domestic services.

This has resulted in a fragmentation of the hospital services and created a need to 'integrate' them in order to provide an effective overall service. Again the service of technology has been sought and there are currently pilot systems aimed at developing an integrated Hospital Information System, which will provide the necessary information and communication links to co-ordinate the specialised units and central services.

Computer-based data processing systems were first developed in hospitals for general administrative purposes - accounts, wages, statistics etc. The next area to be developed was the central service units - for pharmacy management etc. The nursing sector is now beginning to come into contact with computer based information systems, though so far with little direct contact for nursing staff. The nursing process has yet to be computerised.

1.6   The Impact of New Technology on Nurses and Patients

The introduction of new technology is often accompanied by the reorganisation of work. Examples have already been given of increased division of labour and specialisation of skills which accompany technological change. Changes in organisational structure and work organisation also have an impact on staff and patients and thus the analysis of new technology must examine both the indirect impact through organisational change, and the impact as experienced directly.

There is now a substantial amount of research on the social and psychological effects of new technology. Much of this is concerned with the ergonomic aspects of design - creating a match between the person and the machine. The earlier research focused on perceptual-motor skills, but more recently attention has turned to more complex 'cognitive' skills. Some researchers have emphasised the need to design technology to suit the physical, mental and social needs and abilities of its users. Others have concentrated on the need for high quality training in the use of equipment so that users are in a position to work with it competently and confidently. Clearly both good design and training are important, the alternative being ineffective use and stress for the users. This follows from our stress model which indicates that the consequence of an environmental demand which exceeds the resources of the individual is stress.

Working with new technology has brought a qualitative change in the content of work for many people, particularly in those jobs characterised by a high level of skills, for example nursing. Compared with 'traditional' work, working with new technology may be characterised by:

(1)   A shift from manual to intellectual skills.

(2)   A growing distance between the users and the product or process they are working on.

(3)   A shift from concrete, visible targets to more abstract ones.

(4)   Representation of the work process as a mental model that is acted on through intervention and regulation, without the work process necessarily being accesible or directly observable to the user.

(5)   Increasing skill requirements and the need to regularly update skills (Agervold and Kristensen, 1985).

These conclusions are general, and to date there has been little research on the impact on nursing personnel per se. It seems plausible though, that the above factors will apply in particular to nurses using advanced monitoring technology. These 'hypotheses' will be tested in this report.

There is a danger that if nurses come to rely on the monitoring technology, their role could become more passive and this could lead to an atrophy (or de-learning) of conventional powers of observation and nursing skill. If there is an increasing tendency to rely on monitoring equipment to decide when the patient's condition is moving in a dangerous direction, this may in time become the only means of assessment, and the nurse will be dependent on the technology. This 'de-skilling', if it occurred, would have particularly stressful consequences in the event of machine unrelia- bility or breakdown, when a nurse might have difficulty switching from a passive role to active responsibility for patients. Stress itself can have a debilitating effect and make nurses less confident and effective in their intervention and treatment in relation to patients. Alternatively, however, the beneficial effects of the technology may relieve stress for the nurses by supporting them in the provision of patient care.

For the patient, who is the 'object' on which the process control technology is operating, there is a potential danger of becoming more distanced from the nursing staff. Thus any reassurance provided by the technology may be more than off-set by the alienating effects of reduced contract with nurses. The environment of an Intensive Care Unit is likely to be stressful for patients (constant light and noise etc) which might compound their anxious state, inevitably induced by the seriousness of their illness. There is some evidence that Intensive Care Units can be disorientating for conscious patients after a few days, and they can suffer from amnesia (Jones, 1979; Kornfeld, 1969).

Previous research has found that nurses new to intensive care technologies tend to react in one of two ways. They either concentrate on the machines to the exclusion of the patient, or alternatively disregard the machine completely and concentrate on the patient (Yates, 1983).

To avoid some of the difficulties experienced by nurses it seems important that they should be actively involved in the introduction of new technology, and that continued development should take into consideration the experience nurses possess in patient care and the use of the technology (Zielstorff, 1978).

A number of studies have examined nurses and patients attitudes to new technology in medical settings (Cruickshank, 1982, 1984; Hepworth and Fitter, 1981; Potter, 1981; Pringle et al., 1984; Reznikoff et al., 1967; Rosenberg et al., 1967; Startsman and Robinson, 1972). Generally the results indicate that although nurses tend to have more negative attitudes than doctors, direct experience of new technology results in more positive attitudes. Senior nursing staff (management) tend to be more positive than basic grades. Specialist nurses, for example those in Intensive Care Units, are also more positive than nurses on general wards. This may be a consequence of more direct experience of technology generally. There may also be a degree of self selection, nurses inclined towards technology being more likely to work in specialist units.

Similarly patients who have had experience of computer technology, either through personal use or because they had experienced their doctor using one during a consultation, have more positive attitudes to their use in medicine. Also younger and male patients tend to have more positive attitudes.

However previous studies have not examined directly patients' experience of hospital technology and this is one of the aims of this study.

2.0 THE CASE STUDIES

This, the central section of the report, presents in turn the studies carried out in the six European countries. For each study a brief summary is provided of the hospital environment(s), the new technologies in use, and the research methodology of the case study (or studies). This is followed by a presentation of the main findings of the study. The studies have been grouped into sections based on the environments researched. The first five studies all examine the impact of monitoring and treatment technologies in use in high technology environments. The third and fifth studies also examine the use of technology in low technology units. This enables an assessment to be made of the effect of technological complexity on nurses and their work. The sixth study looks at the use of a Management Information System as it affects a group of units organised into a single department.

2.1 New Technology in Intensive Care Units

An Intensive Care Unit accommodates patients who need constant monitoring of certain physiological functions, on account of the high risk of death that exists for these patients. This constrains the type of work organisation that can exist in the unit. The patients are linked to equipment which keeps a check on vital functions and are observed for 24 hours a day by a medical and nursing team. Patients will sometimes be in one large central room so that all beds can be observed from a single point, or will be separated into single rooms or cubicles if the technology allows remote monitoring and/or there is sufficient nursing staff on duty to observe each bed. Most nursing staff are required to work a three shift system to provide the necessary 24 hour cover.

The technology may be divided into monitoring equipment and support equipment.

The principal types of monitoring equipment record and display on a screen, for ease of reading by the doctor and nurse, the following variables:

(1)   The electrocardiograph trace, with indication of heart-rate.
(2)   Arterial and/or vein pressure.

(3)   The electroencephalograph trace.

(4)   The carbon dioxide level in the blood, to help in evaluating respiratory alkalosis and acidosis.

These recordings are partly non-invasive, as in the use of surface electrodes to record the ECG and EEG trace, and partly invasive, as in the case of recording pressure in the arteries and veins by means of a device inserted into an artery or vein.

All monitoring devices are nowadays, in the most modern equipment, grouped together into a single small machine which displays the data in easily-read forms, either digital or graphic, on a screen. Patients can be linked, during the period of hospitalisation in the Unit, to this kind of machine which sets off an acoustic alarm whenever the physiological indicators go outside their pre-set limits.

The support equipment is designed to facilitate and reactivate vital physiological functions. Commonly used machines include:

(1)   The automatic breathing machine, which is used to facilitate or maintain this function. The tube may be of two different types: nasal-tracheal when it is inserted through the nose, or endotracheal when the patient undergoes a tracheotomy.

(2)   The oxygen humidifier, which is applied to the patient's face through a mask.

(3)   The defibrillator, an instrument which is used to interrupt fibrillation of the heart if it should occur.

The equipment used in the unit could also usefully be classified, for the purposes of the present report, into invasive and non-invasive equipment.

Examples of invasive equipment would include automatic nasaltracheal and endotrachael respirators, and also the pressure measurement devices which are inserted by means of needles into the arteries and veins of the patient. The oxygen humidifier, although it is not an invasive instrument, is in effect highly upsetting to conscious patients.

2.2   The Danish Study

The Danish Report focuses on the impact of computer-based patient monitoring technology, used in a coronary care ward of a large University hospital.

2.2.1   The environment

The hospital in Aarhus has, in total, some 1,400 beds and employes over 2,000 permanent staff engaged in patient care. Of these some 1,400 are nurses.

The ward is an intensive care monitoring and post treatment ward for coronary patients. It has 22 beds: 16-18 cardiac-medical beds and four cardiac-surgery beds. The ward consists of two sections, a primary section with six single rooms and one twin room, all with special equipment for monitoring heart functions, and a secondary section consisting of two bedded rooms without fixed monitoring equipment, but with facilities for radio monitoring (telemetry).

The average length of stay for patients is 6.7 days, this is a substantial decrease from the 1981 duration of 8.4 days. The medical staff in B Block, which also includes the cardiological laboratory and a second ward, consists of four consultants, five senior registrars, eight registrars, a clinical assistant and 32 nurses (27 female, 5 male). Two of the nurses are on permanent night duty, five work part-time on permanent evening duty and the remaining 27 work rotating shifts. Shiftwork involves about 10 evening and night duties per month and working every other weekend. The duty schedule is prepared for a month by two nurses in turn, and there is a book where nurses can record a month in advance requests for special days off etc. The schedule requires at least nine nurses on duty in the daytime, five in the evening and four at night. The nursing administration describe absenteeism through illness as relatively low (about 25%, which is about the hospital average). However, staff turnover is fairly high, the average stay being 1½ to 3 years.

The form of nursing in the ward is assigned patient care, where the objective is that patients are nursed by the same staff throughout their stay on the ward. This is to counteract lack of continuity and alienation in nursing, and encourage the patients and their relatives to be jointly responsible and active in the recovery process. The ward has no fixed visiting hours, and there is a room for relatives in the ward, which also has facilities for them to stay overnight. Assigned patient nursing involves a fairly high degree of autonomy for nurses, and is based on a 'flattened' management structure in which the ward sister's role is primarily that of a co-ordinator.

The nurses' responsibilities for patient care include referral for treatment to specialist departments, care, hygiene, administration of medication, and treatment for cardiac arrest. The job also includes varying amounts of clerical work, and specific responsibilities for the monitoring technology, viz recording a sample ECG trace for each of their assigned patients to check the signal's nature; keeping a constant eye for atypical heartrates; collecting ECG recordings with unusual characteristics for the case-file. The nurses are also responsible for checking and maintaining the central monitoring equipment and the equipment in the patient's room, including the electrodes.

2.2.2 The technologies

The monitoring system in the coronary care ward is Hewlett Packard's Arrhythmia computer system HP78525, the main purpose of which is to identify abnormal deflections on the individual ECG curves recorded on the machine for each patient in order to commence intervention and treatment as rapidly as possible. It was installed in 1980 when the ward moved from an old building to its current new one.

The monitoring system covers two types of supervision:

(1)   In 10 single rooms for acute patients, transmission of electrode signals to an oscilloscope by the bed, and transmission to the display unit in the central monitoring room

(2)   Six telemetric monitoring sets, by which electrode signals are transmitted via radio antennae to the display unit in the central monitoring room. This makes it possible for patients to move freely around the ward.

ECG information is stored in the computer for up to 24 hours, and a printer is used to produce trend curves and histograms, collate alarms, and summarise individual patients' ECG records. The monitoring system includes three types of alarm:

*   Red: to indicate ventricle fibrillation, cardiac arrest, ventricular tachycardia and extreme bradycardia. It is activated either automatically as a result of computer detection or manually by a nurse in the patient's room. The red alarm lights a red lamp outside the room and a sound alarm in the corridor and the control rooms.
*   Yellow: to indicate that the lower or upper limits for heart-rate have been exceeded. A lamp lights in the control room indicating the source, a sound alarm emits for 5 seconds, and the printer produces a strip of ECG to reveal the cause of the alarm.
*   Green: no sound alarm is activated, nor is there a printout, but green lamps light in the monitoring room.

For all types of alarm the first action of the nursing staff is to go to the control room and examine the ECG trace to see if the alarm is false. This is done because many alarms (up to 50%) are false and the nurses wish to avoid going into the patient's room and causing stress by checking more often than is absolutely necessary.

2.2.3 The research methodology

The study involved interviewing all 32 nurses working on the ward. Topics addressed included job content, satisfaction, training and use of technology, stressors and coping responses. A psychological and psychosomatic reactions questionnaire was completed by all nurses. The 27 full-time nurses also completed a daily diary of work descriptions and stress reactions at the end of their shift.

The interviews were the main source of the data collection (each interview had a duration of about one hour) and the scoring procedure was done independently by both the investigators, and then they agreed a score on each variable for each nurse. From these measures each nurse was categorised into one of three groups: low, medium and high functioning in the 15 variables subdivided into two main independent groups: (a) organisational factors: shiftwork and quality of working life, and (b) technology: qualifications, attitudes, breakdowns, alarms etc. In the further analysis the independent variables were related to the dependant variables: six variables covering coping and health, partly based on a checklist of the prevalence of psychic and psychosomatic complaints.

As a supplement to these data, a daily checklist of perceived stress (on a 5-point scale) was used to indicate whether nurses currently had any of the following symptoms: headache, muscle pain in the upper or lower back, pains in the legs, tired eyes, physical or mental fatigue; and finally the working day was rated on the basis of ten different stressors (e.g. problems with colleagues, superiors, patients, patients' relatives, and technology). Each stressful circumstance was scored between 0 and 3, so the total stress rating for a shift could vary between 0 and 30.

The study also gathered information through direct observations on the ward, by interviews with doctors and relevant experts, and by the examination of written material.

Finally a sample of 10 patients were interviewed upon discharge from the ward about their perceptions of the ward and the technology in use.

2.2.4 The research findings

Job characteristics and stressors:

The study confirmed the presence of many of the work environment stressors that have been found in other hospital studies and have been reviewed in the introduction. Specifically it was found that:

(1)   Stress is created by the high work pace, and this combined with

(2)   Cognitive demands relating, on the one hand, to nursing and treat-ment related assessments and decisions of a more complex nature and, on the other hand, to analysis, assessment and interpretation of the information from the monitoring equipment.

(3)   Interaction with seriously ill patients and their relatives is stressful, as is

(4)   Shiftwork involving a heavy burden of turns on duty.

(5)   Working with the monitoring technology when a high incidence of alarms occurs - particularly false ones - makes severe demands on the nurse.

These stressors are compensated for by other job factors which are mainly positive:

(1)   The quality of work, including job characteristics such as the degree of variation, responsibility, interest and independence, the scope for personal and cognitive development, and the importance and significance perceived by patients and relatives.
(2)   Training and skill enhancing opportunities.
(3)   Relations with colleagues and superiors in a good and open climate of co-operation.
(4)   Good opportunities for social support and help from colleagues and superiors in difficult work situations.

From a total of 102 observation periods reports from 19 nurses across all shifts revealed that the most stressful work circumstances which occur most frequently are the high pace and situations which call for difficult decisions in relation to patients and their treatment, and only to a lesser degree are there problems in connection with the technology.

Stress experienced:

The stressors combine to produce a total effect in the form of stress experienced by each individual. The picture that emerges of general stress reactions is that there are frequent incidents of mental fatigue or short-term stress, and many nurses also report psychological stress symptoms. However, the incidence of psychosomatic stress does not appear to be very pronounced, and similarly absenteeism through illness is at the level found in other wards.

The sub-division of nurses into low and high functioning groups revealed some interesting differences in the self reported stress reactions, as are illustrated in tables 2.2.1 and 2.2.2.

Table 2.2.1 indicates that the low-functioning group is characterised by female nurses who have relatively little experience on the ward and who are less likely to have had previous experience of working with new technology.

Table 2.2.1:
Distribution of personal variables between low, medium and high functioning groups

| | Sex: Number of | | Age (yrs) | Experience in the ward (yrs) | Worked previously with new technology |
	Women	Men			
Low functioning group	8	0	29.4	1.7	38%
Med functioning group	14	3	30.9	2.9	47%
High functioning group	5	2	31.9	4.4	71%
Average	27	5	30.7	3.0	50%

Table 2.2.2:
Distribution of psychological stress variables between low, medium and high functioning groups. Scale variations from -2 to +2

	N	Perceived Social support	Action and coping strategies	Burn-out	Mental fatigue	Psychological stress	Psychosomatic stress
Low functioning group	8	0.75	-1.00	-0.75	-1.63	-1.25	-0.88
Med functioning group	17	1.47	-0.24	0.24	-0.82	-0.35	0.24
High functioning group	7	1.71	0.57	0.57	0.14	0.57	1.43
Average	32	1.31	-0.22	0.02	-0.77	-0.34	0.26

Supports and coping strategies:

Table 2.2.2 presents some of the support, coping and stress variables. It reveals that the low-functioning group have less social support available, and see less opportunities for remedial action to reduce stress. It was also found that the low-functioning group was more likely to report individual strategies for coping with stress e.g. talking with colleagues/ families, taking exercise and undergoing therapy etc. However an individual strategy may be less effective than the possibility of group action to change the source of stress because the low-functioning group experienced higher levels of burn-out, mental fatigue, and psychological and psychosomatic stress as illustrated in table 2.2.2. The low-functioning group also found the training less adequate and wanted more than the other groups. There is some evidence that the 'assigned' method of nursing may lead to a feeling of isolation from colleagues for some of the nurses in this group. These results are summarised in figure 2.2.1

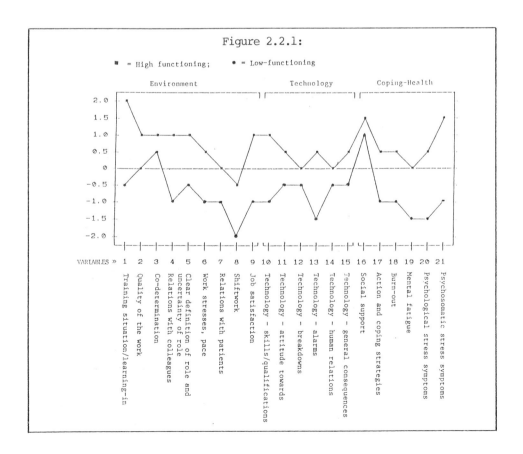

Figure 2.2.1:

To make the differences between the two functional groups more explicit, two "average persons" from the high- and low-functioning groups respectively have been constructed.

Figure 2.2.1 shows a clear difference in level for these average persons, which is again to be found for all variables. The results therefore reinforce the theoretical hypothesis that there is a connection between the way in which a person functions in a given work environment and his well-being from a health aspect, since there appear to be clear connections between a work-functional level and a health-functional level.

The impact of new technology on the nurses:

All the nurses but one regard the monitoring technology as an aid to their work - a safety net that gives them a certain amount of freedom. The two main advantages of the monitoring technology in relation to patients and nursing are seen as:

(1)   The monitoring system makes rapid medical and treatment intervention possible and thereby ensures maximum treatment.
(2)   The monitoring system eases the nurses' work, since it continuously observes changes in the heart rate. It also records conditions that may be invisible to the nurses' clinical observation.

However, one in three nurses also perceive the monitoring technology as straining their relationship with patients, since there is a tendency to keep staring at the equipment at the expense of the actual care of patients. Some patients become pre-occupied by the heart rate on the screen. Thus the technology can have an alienating effect on relations between nurse and patient. Other disadvantages for the patient reported by nurses include a risk of isolation because nurses visit their rooms less often, noise from equipment, and at times the frequent need to disturb the patient for checking electrodes, measuring blood pressure etc. If the nurse notices something on the screen which the patient is not aware of she/he must be careful not to alarm the patient. A few of the nurses view the monitoring equipment as giving them closer contact with the patients.

Training in the use of the monitoring technology is mainly carried out by the nurses themselves - skills are passed on to new recruits and it takes at least a year to feel adequately qualified. This places a burden on the experienced nurses, which can be stressful, because the relatively high turnover on the ward means that training is a continual process.

Over half the nurses are dissatisfied with the training programme for introducing the monitoring technology (the ward's doctors provide two 16 hour courses per year on the observation and treatment of coronary patients). The remainder are satisfied and emphasise that it is the responsibility of the individual to acquire the necessary knowledge and skills through practice and support from colleagues. Commitment and interest is crucial if nurses are to develop an adequate understanding of the technology. The nurses regard the learning process as unending, particularly on the interpretation of heart rate and cardiac arrhythmias. It is common for nurses to seek help in interpretation from one another and from the doctors.

As well as helping them, the nurses see the technology also as a stressor, and views fall into three main categories:

(1)   The interpretation and assessment of information provided by the equipment is a cognitive stress. This is particularly the case when sitting in the control room monitoring several screens simultaneously.

(2)   The alarm system is an important element of the monitoring installation, and it is also the one part of the monitoring system that all nurses say is seriously stressful because of the frequent and inaccurate alarms. But although everyone perceived frequent alarms as a stress, the justification for their existence is not contested, neither is their nature as a support in the work. This supportive function of the alarms is acknowledged by four out of five nurses. Assessment of whether an alarm is true or false, and thus whether it demands action, is obviously a matter of experience. For example, only the youngest nurses say that they find this assessment stressful, whereas the great majority – more than two thirds – find that with experience it is relatively uncomplicated. Nevertheless the over-stimulation caused by the frequent alarms leads to a cognitive 'switching-off'. This defensive coping strategy is reported to have possible damaging longer-term consequences for the nurses' self-image and professional pride.

"It has not taken over any of my skills, because you can't rely on
it entirely. You must be able to do most things yourself."

Most nurses report the technology as having no overall effect on the
quality of their work, though one in four see it as having a negative
effect. Similarly the majority see it as having no overall effect on job
satisfaction, the positive effects as an aid being countered by the stress
of false alarms and the tendency for nurse and patient to become pre-
occupied with the screens.

The patients' views:

All patients interviewed had positive views about the ward, the staff and
the care they had received:

"It's wonderful to be in a place where you're in able hands. This
is the most important thing when you're in hospital.

Most patients do not remember much about admission, at the time they are
usually unconscious or confused by pain or pain-killing drugs. Their
perception of the equipment once they regain consciousness is often contradictory. On the one hand they find it reassuring, on the other, they see
it as an alienating element in their situation.

"You get a bit frightened when you wake up and see all the instruments and apparatus connected to you. And you think, is it all this
or yourself that will be controlling your body - but you soon get
over it ..."

The ideology that prevails in the ward promotes the active participation of
patients in the procedures involved in their recovery. This is difficult
with the monitoring technology which reduces patient involvement to a
minimum and is perceived as having a pacifying effect:

"I felt completely safe while I was being monitored; the moment the
slightest thing happened they came rushing in to see what was the
matter. I felt absolutely certain that they would look after me,
and therefore I didn't have to do anything myself."

(3)   The monitoring technology 'demands' a response. The availability of
       resuscitation equipment makes it possible to deal with a cardiac
       arrest. The nurses therefore feel <u>obliged</u> to respond in all circum-
       stances. This can at times conflict with their own views on the
       ethical desirability of resuscitation. There are frequent discus-
       sions amongst nurses and with doctors who have the responsibility
       for the decision. Even though it is the doctors' decision, the
       considerations are prominent in the nurses' thinking and promote
       feelings of stress.

A severe stress factor in working with the monitoring equipment is when it
breaks down. Two-thirds of the nurses report it as stressful. The extent
of the stress varies, experienced nurses can take it in their stride
whereas inexperienced nurses can be very concerned, for example:

> "I've experienced a breakdown and it was dreadful. The alarm kept
> on going and it spat out paper. It howled along the whole corridor,
> and people are fully aware that when it howls something is <u>really</u>
> wrong. Of course it also affected us - and we couldn't make it
> stop. Also, it takes a frightful time to connect up all the alarms
> again, and if you have to do this at a time when you're really busy
> it's very stressful. It's also hectic and confusing when suddenly
> no patients are being monitored any more - you feel helpless; how
> are the patients? You have to think for yourself ..."

Only the more experienced nurses know how to restart after a breakdown, two
out of three nurses saying they do not know how to. However, this does not
mean they are at a complete loss because they can refer to the operating
manual if necessary.

One in three nurses see the technology as having a negative effect on co-
operation. This is mainly the younger nurses who feel dependent on the
more experienced ones and sometimes feel they are regarded as stupid. The
other two-thirds report the technology as having no effect on co-operation.

Only one in four nurses regard the technology as taking over their
functions and skills. The remainder see it as an <u>aid</u> to patient
monitoring, but with decisions still made by the nurses:

The view of some of the nurses that they and the patients tend to become pre-occupied with the screens is also the view of some patients:

> "I sit about a lot looking at the 'scope, keeping an eye on how my heart is beating. It can make you quite crazy ..."

Although it is perhaps debatable whether patients relinquishing responsibility for their recovery actually inhibits the healing process or not, the view that they should be passive was quite common among patients:

> "I don't ask very much about my illness. I'm content with short answers. I take it for granted that what they say is right. My view is that this thing with my heart is their affair, and I don't interfere. Let them do what they know how to do. Those officious patients must be irritating for the doctors."

One way of dealing with these issues of passivity and responsibility is for nurses and patients to have more time to talk together. However both nurses and patients see the nurses as too busy to have the time necessary for more than essential contact.

2.2.5 Overview of the study

The Danish study has focused on the impact of a computer-based patient monitoring system in a coronary care unit. The study combined interview data and established questionnaires to assess nurses' psychological and psychosomatic stress reactions. Nurses also kept daily work descriptions and recorded their stress reactions at the end of each shift. The data was used to categorise the 32 nurses into three sub-groups (low, medium and high functioning) based on their level of reported stress.

The study confirmed the presence of many of the work environment stressors that have been found in previous hospital studies, in particular the high pace of work, complex cognitive demands, dealing with seriously ill patients and their relatives, shiftwork, and working with unreliable technology. Job factors which compensated for these stressors were the importance of the work combined with a high degree of responsibility, and job variety, and opportunity to use skills. There was also a high level of support from colleagues and superiors, and a climate of co-operation. The low functioning group of nurses contained a predominance of younger nurses with little previous experience of working with new technology. These nurses were also more likely to report individual strategies for coping with stress (such as unwinding after work), though such strategies were seen as less effective than dealing with the source of stress by attempting to influence the work environment. The 'assigned' method of nursing, which paired patient and nurse for a shift, was also seen as reducing the need for contact between nurses and contributing to the isolation experienced by some of the nurses in this group.

Almost all the nurses regarded the monitoring technology as an aid to their work - a safety net that gave them a certain amount of freedom. However, some nurses also saw it as straining their relationship with the patients because of its tendency to distract them from direct communication. Training in use of the technology was mainly carried out by the nurses themselves passing on their skills. It was estimated that it took at least a year to feel adequately qualified, and over half the nurses felt dissatisfied with the training programme.

The technology was seen as a source of stress because of the cognitive demands and the need for a rapid response to alarms. There were a high proportion of false alarms which were particularly stressful as were equipment breakdowns.

The majority of nurses reported that the technology had no overall effect on the quality of their work, or on job satisfaction because the positive effects of the aid were cancelled by the stress of false alarms, and the tendency to become pre-occupied with the monitors.

All patients had positive views about the ward and its staff. They tended to have contradictory views about the technology, in part seeing it as necessary and reassuring, but also finding it a bit frightening and alienating. There is a policy on the ward of promoting the active participation of patients in their recovery. There was concern that some patients either became pre-occupied with the monitors measuring their own vital functions, or felt they should adopt a completely passive role in the hands of the staff and the technology.

2.3   The Irish Study

The Irish report examines the impact of new technology in high technology Units in five hospitals in the Dublin area. The study focuses on the work experiences and stressors; in particular those relating to new technology in a sample of 52 nurses in a range of work environments.

2.3.1   The environments

In three of the five hospitals (A, B and C) Intensive Care and Coronary Care Units were studied. The other two hospitals (D and E) provide maternity services and the study focused on the Neonatal Intensive Care Units. Although observations and interviews were conducted in all five hospitals an analysis of the work environment was not made in hospital E. A description of the environment in the Units studied in the four hospitals is provided below:

Hospital A:

Two wards were studied in this 280 bed nineteenth century city centre hospital with approximately 213 qualified and 245 student nurses. A particular feature of the hospital is that Units are spread over a wide area and this creates problems transporting patients and conveying information and test materials, supplies, etc over large distances.

The Coronary Care ward has five beds for pre and post operative patients. Thirteen staff nurses and a ward sister work on the ward, with a three shift system operated on a five week cycle (three weeks of days, one of nights and one week off). The morning shift has three nurses, and the afternoon/evening and night shifts each have two nurses on duty. Nursing turnover is relatively high, with an average stay of six to twelve months. Patients stay in the ward for on average 3 days, with a bed occupancy of a little over 80%.

The Intensive Care Unit has four beds, separated into individual cubicles, and is staffed by 20 nurses and a ward sister. The shift system is the same as for the Coronary Unit, with four nurses on morning shift, three on afternoon/evening, and two on nights. Nursing turnover is relatively low, with a stay of some two to ten years. Patients stay in the ward for between three days and three weeks.

Hospital B:

Two Units were studied in this old 456 bed city centre hospital with approximately 280 qualified and 300 student nurses. A new complex is being built for the hospital. Although nurses' experiences were assessed in the Intensive Care Unit and the Coronary Care Units, the environment of only the former was assessed.

The Intensive Care Unit has 10 beds and 40 nursing personnel, composed of five sisters, 10 staff nurses with expert experience, 10 staff nurses with moderate experience, and 10 junior staff nurses. There are also approximately eight post-graduate Intensive Care trainees. The shift rotas are compiled so as to balance the skills available on each shift. This procedure was introduced six months previously and is regarded as resulting in a major reduction in stress.

The five week cycle shift system consists of three weeks of days, a week of nights and a week off. In each week of days, one of the days is a long shift of $13\frac{1}{4}$ hours and this is regarded by nurses as particularly difficult. Nursing turnover is relatively low, nurses staying up to 10 years. Patient stays are very short, each bed being occupied by three patients per week on average.

Hospital C:

This is also a nineteenth century city centre hospital and has 194 beds with approximately 70 qualified and 97 student nurses. The Units studied were the Intensive Care Unit with three beds, and the Coronary Care Unit with six beds. There are 25 beds in the section which contains these two Units, it has 27 staff nurses plus one student. Although on a shift nurses are assigned to one Unit, they are located in a central station which overlooks both Units. It is accepted that nurses help out in the other Unit if requested. Again it is important that each shift balances the level of experience available. The shift system is similar to that of Hospital A, except that for one week of the cycle there is a split day shift, which is very unpopular amongst nursing staff. Yet nursing turnover is relatively low, many having seven or eight years experience in ICU/CCU. The flexibility of the job rotation between Units is seen as positive and it is described as a means of reducing stress.

A pastoral care service to support seriously ill and dying patients is provided in the Units by a trained volunteer. This counselling service is regarded as a benefit by both patients and nurses.

Hospital D:

This is a 243 bed nineteenth century maternity hospital with 140 qualified (in midwifery) nurses and 100 students. Approximately 40 babies are in the Neonatal section, of who some 20 are in the seriously ill category. The study focuses on this part, the Neonatal Intensive Care Unit which has 50% nursing staff who have a special training in NIC, and 50% who are qualified nurses being trained in NIC. The hospital has been foremost in promoting training in Neonatal Intensive Care. The shift system is similar to that in Hospital A, and for each shift two qualified nurses are always on duty.

The work environment in the Unit is a source of stress for staff since it is hot (78°F), and the conditions are cramped, and there is a continual glare from the lights. The blue lights in the Phototherapy Unit are regarded as particularly stressful.

2.3.2   The technologies

A considerable variety of equipment is in use in the range of Units examined by the Irish case study. Some of the equipment is in regular use in a Unit (core equipment), and other is used only infrequently and for particular cases (special equipment). Table 2.3.1 list the technology in use, as described in questionnaires by nurses in each of the environments studied.

```
┌────────────────────────────────────────────────────────────────────┐
│                          Table 2.3.1:                                │
│             Core technology and special technology used in           │
│            intensive care, coronary care and neonatal care           │
│                                                                      │
│  Type of Unit            Core equipment          Special equipment   │
│  1  Intensive care       Ventilator              Intra Aortic Pump   │
│                          Defibrilator            Hewlett Packard      │
│                          Cardiac Monitor         Haemodynamic Monitor │
│                          Space Lab Monitor       Dialysis            │
│                          IVAC - Drips            Swan Ganz           │
│                          ECG                     Cardiac Output      │
│                                                  Infusion Pump       │
│  2  Coronary care        Ventilator              ECG                 │
│                          Respirator              Swan Ganz           │
│                          Defibrilator            Cardiac Output      │
│                          Cardiac Monitor                             │
│                          Central Monitor                             │
│                          Space Lab Monitor                           │
│                          IVAC - Drips                                │
│  3  Neonatal care        Ventilator              Resuscitation Equipment │
│                          Cardiac Monitor         Transport Monitors  │
│                          Apnoea Monitor                              │
│                          Space Lab Monitor                           │
│                          TCPO2 Monitor                               │
│                          Incubators                                  │
└────────────────────────────────────────────────────────────────────┘
```

Type of Unit	Core equipment	Special equipment
1 Intensive care	Ventilator	Intra Aortic Pump
	Defibrilator	Hewlett Packard
	Cardiac Monitor	Haemodynamic Monitor
	Space Lab Monitor	Dialysis
	IVAC - Drips	Swan Ganz
	ECG	Cardiac Output
		Infusion Pump
2 Coronary care	Ventilator	ECG
	Respirator	Swan Ganz
	Defibrilator	Cardiac Output
	Cardiac Monitor	
	Central Monitor	
	Space Lab Monitor	
	IVAC - Drips	
3 Neonatal care	Ventilator	Resuscitation Equipment
	Cardiac Monitor	Transport Monitors
	Apnoea Monitor	
	Space Lab Monitor	
	TCPO2 Monitor	
	Incubators	

2.3.3 The research methodology

Case studies were carried out in Intensive and Coronary Care Units in three
of the hospitals. These involved observation of work activities, and in
depth interviews with nursing staff about their work, the technologies in
use, training received, and the demands of technology and skills required.
Views of equipment suppliers, especially concerning their role in training
and maintenance, were also obtained. Fifteen experts (matrons, heads of
nursing and training schools, nurse tutors and physiotherapists) were also
interviewed, as well as 12 nurses as a preliminary to the in depth case
studies.

A second component to the study involved the completion of a range of questionnaires by 52 ward sisters and nurses in the five hospitals studied:

Hospital A:	9 nurses (ICU and CCU)
Hospital B:	13 nurses (ICU and CCU)
Hospital C:	10 nurses (ICU and CCU)
Hospitals D and E:	20 nurses (neonatal)

Questions to nurses concerned attitudes to, and perceptions of (a) their job, (b) new technology, (c) stress, and (d) coping behaviour. Special attitude scales were developed to measure the main variables in the study, with the exception of a measure of anxiety which was an established scale (Spielberger et al., 1970).

Finally a sample of 18 patients who had been in an Intensive or Coronary Care Unit responded to a questionnaire concerning their attitudes towards and perceptions of new technology in the Unit.

2.3.4 The research findings

Job characteristics and stressors:

The study confirmed the presence of several of the environmental stressors previously reported. When nurses were asked to rank order nine job related factors (based on the work of Claus, Bailey and Selye, 1980) by the extent to which they induced stress, the rank ordering reported was as follows (most stressful first):

(1)   Organisation of the Unit (lack of time, shift schedules, inadequate staffing).

(2)   Inadequate skill and knowledge (lack of experience and skill, unfamiliar situation, lack of knowledge).

(3)   Interpersonal conflict (conflicts between members of the work team).

(4)   Patient care (emergencies, critically ill, unstable patients, death and dying of special patients, uncooperative patients, routine procedures).

(5)   Performance and use of skills (a sense of knowledge and skills, handling emergencies, anticipating situations).

(6)   Physical work environment (work space, noise, heat, too many people).

(7)   Acquisition of knowledge (learning techniques and theory, intellectual challenge).

(8)   Reward system at work (pay, benefits, promotion, opportunity).

(9)   ICU-CCU environment (challenge, variety, excitement, pace).

The most pronounced of these stressors do not relate directly to new technology per se, but are a consequence of the high pressure of work which is characteristic of Intensive Care Units and the emotional pressure of working with critically ill and dying ptients. The perceived lack of knowledge and skill is perhaps a consequence of the relatively high proportion of unqualified or partially qualified staff in the units (this factor is reported as partially ameliorated recently by the balancing of shifts so they contain a cross section of skill levels). There also appears to be a considerable level of interpersonal conflict perceived in the units and 'lack of teamwork' emerged as a major stressor. The organisational climate (measured on a 12-item scale; McCarthy, 1979) is a particular source of pressure and strain to a substantial percentage of employees. These are not general characteristics of work in Intensive Care Units, for example, the hospital has a lot of bureaucratic regulations and is not seen as supportive by 56% of nurses. Lack of knowledge and lack of interpersonal support were not seen as major stressors in the Danish study, which found that interpersonal support was a positive job factor.

In the Irish study nurses perceived the main positive aspect of their job as its meaningfulness and contribution to society. Although shiftwork was generally seen positively, the split-day and long-day (12 or 13 hours) shifts were not liked.

Supports and coping strategies:

Nurses reported that they coped with stress by unwinding off-the-job. That is, the major source of coping was external to the job, and even here 47% of nurses reported difficulty unwinding. In particular, a correlational analysis of the data indicated that nurses who were more 'care' oriented also needed to unwind more after work.

The alternative means of coping with stress (<u>internal</u> mechanisms such as feeling competent and able to control or limit stressors), was reported by some nurses, but did not appear to be particularly effective in these Units. This is consistent with a perceived low degree of control, stressful organisation and lack of team support. Thus it appears that, to a significant extent, nurses had to use their own 'free' time to handle the effects of stressors rather than deal with them in the workplace itself.

<u>The impact of new technology on the nurses</u>:

A number of questionnaire items directly assessed the impact of new technology. The picture emerges that the majority of nurses view new technology as helpful in their Units, enabling them to do a good job. However more specific questions indicate nurses' concern about their using the technology, and the extent to which it takes their attention away from the patient.

A 15 item questionnaire scale was used to examine nurses' perceptions of stress created by the technology. The items focused on:

(a)   Machine demands and anxiety.
(b)   Combining machine monitoring with patient monitoring.
(c)   Cognitive aspects of machine handling.

The items were rated on a four point scale (1 = no stress to 4 = considerable stress). Table 2.3.2 shows the five items which were reported as causing the greatest stress, each having a score of more than 2.0

It is apparent that equipment reliability is a major source of stress for the nurses. This is indicated by items 1 (poor maintenance) and 4 (break-downs) in table 2.3.2. This finding is similar to a finding of the Danish study in which false alarms with the equipment were a major stressor. Nurses reported that not everyone had the same understanding of the functions and uses of the equipment and this could lead to mistakes. Equipment sometimes appears to break down because of the large number of staff handling it.

Table 2.3.2:

The top five technology stressors reported by
52 nurses, the mean score for the item (four point scale)
and the percentage of nurses reporting 'considerable stress'

Item	Mean Score	% 'considerable 'stress'
1 Poor maintenance of machines	2.69	35
2 Not having sufficient understanding of how key pieces of equipment work	2.72	21
3 Spending too much time and energy with the technology and not giving enough time to talking to and supporting the patient	2.68	14
4 Breakdown of machine	2.58	21
5 Handling all the technology and life-support machines effectively for each patient	2.27	12

Problems are seen to arise because of inadequate consultation with nursing staff over the acquisition of equipment even though they are the principal users. This varies from hospital to hospital. In Hospital A the advice of nurses was not sought when equipment was installed. The nurses found this frustrating since they felt many simple problems with the technology could be overcome or avoided if use was made of their knowledge and expertise. Hospitals B and C had a policy of involving senior nursing staff in decisions about technology, and the level of satisfaction with it was higher in these hospitals.

Although the new technology was seen as enhancing nurses skills the demands placed on nurses by its use were a major source of stress (items 2 and 5). 45% of nurses indicated they were dissatisfied with the training they received. Training provided by the hospitals was mainly on the job, consisting of either special training in the Unit, or learning by experience. Only a quarter of nurses attended off-the-job courses. Nurses indicated that they had difficulty getting leave of absence to attend recognised courses, since the Department of Health did not make any provision for such training or recognise it as in-service training. It was agreed that training provided by equipment suppliers, whether through demonstrations or through instruction manuals, was inadequate for the specialist work nurses in intensive care have to perform. Moreover nurses had insufficient time to learn from suppliers' demonstrations. The supplier's primary goal is to sell the equipment to the hospitals, though it does have responsibility to ensure that the users of new equipment have become skilled in its use. However, it is the hospital organisation that needs to recognise that learning and training takes time, and that in the long run such training is likely to reduce stress arising from inadequate knowledge, and from working with colleagues who are inexperienced in the use of new technology. With no specialist training provided, trainee nurses learn about the technology informally, and indicated that they felt fearful of using the equipment. These concerns are very real and frightening when nurses are dealing with seriously ill patients. Because of the inadequate training there is a concern that through insufficient understanding of the detailed functioning of the technology nurses may become too dependent on it. A principal fear behind the criticisms of the training appears to be the serious consequences that lack of understanding of life sustaining equipment can have on the patient, and on the erosion of traditional nursing skills.

The third major source of stress was that involvement with the technology took time away from relating to the patient (table 2.3.2, item 3). Moreover 77% of nurses perceived their work as becoming more impersonal because of new technology, and 69% agreed that 'they have become a technician because of new technology rather than a carer'.

More specific probing of nurses' views suggested that nurses see the technology as having a mediating effect between themselves and the patient (71% indicating that the technology had distanced them from the patient). However, 79% of nurses also agreed that 'you cannot differentiate between technical and non-technical aspects of the job - they both serve to care for the patient'. It seems that rather than usurping their role, technology is seen as part of that caring role.

It was striking from observational work in one of the Units that nurses appeared to compensate for a reduction in personal contact by continually talking to patients who were apparently unconscious. Nurses viewed the new technology as potentially intrusive and liable to cause patients considerable distress and anxiety. Once patients demonstrate that they can resume physiological functioning without the aid of machines they are disconnected. Nurses base their observation of patient distress on the physiological and emotional cues which patients display while attached to the equipment. In the view of some nurses, equipment is used in some cases for no clear reason, particularly in the case of equipment which is not life sustaining. When its use cannot be justified on medical grounds they feel it should be abandoned in favour of the patient's psychological welfare.

New technology highlights some ethical dilemmas for nurses. It creates the possibility of prolonging the patient's life but perhaps at a cost of a lower quality life since more patients are surviving who would have previously died. This is particularly the case for babies in the Neonatal Unit who may have sustained brain damage. These concerns raise questions for the nurses about the desirability of maintaining a patient on a machine if there is little chance of recovery. They are also concerned about when to turn a machine off, particularly if there is another patient who could perhaps be better helped by the availability of a scarce resource. These dilemmas are an additional source of stress for staff in high technology units.

The patients' views:

Patients' views were assessed through a questionnaire administered to a sample of 18 who had received coronary care. For 89% of them their general level of anxiety regarding the technology was low. More detailed probing revealed an overall positive perception of new technology used in their diagnosis or treatment while in hospital. They expressed a high degree of confidence in the nurses' abilities and use of technology. They did not generally experience any feelings of alienation from the nurses because of the technology, although they did see the technology as placing an additional burden on the nurses, whom they saw as insufficiently rewarded for their specialist work. While 50% reported a feeling of dependency on the technology, 93% indicated they were grateful it was available for coronary treatment.

Hospital B provides a pastoral care service to support seriously ill and dying patients. A volunteer trained in pastoral care visits and is on call for counselling support to patients and nurses. This service was seen as a benefit to nurses and patients. It was also seen as important that patients be treated as 'cognitive feeling beings' and where practical given some pre-operative advice to prepare them for the changes that will occur. This was seen as reducing anxiety levels and speeding up recovery. Linked to this, a post-operative rehabilitation programme was seen as important. Such a programme is available in Hospital A and is planned for Hospital B.

2.3.5 Overview of the study

The Irish study has used a range of questionnaires and other techniques to examine nurses' views of their work, stressors, and new technology in five hospitals in the Dublin area. A major stressor perceived by nursing staff is the way that their work is organised, which results in a high pace of work and time pressure, and a lack of staff with the necessary skills. The work environment is not seen as supportive and there is a reported lack of teamwork. The main means of coping with stress is to 'unwind' after work, since nurses perceive only limited opportunity to influence the sources of stress in the workplace. Although they regard their work as meaningful and important, they feel they do not get sufficient recognition for it.

New technology is seen as generally a useful and necessary part of nursing work, requiring additional skills for effective and confident operation. However there is a widespread view that the training available is inadequate and therefore the technology is a source of stress because of insufficient knowledge. Training, other than that available from equipment suppliers, is seen as necessary and important.

These problems are exacerbated by breakdowns and problems with the maintenance of the equipment, and because nurses are sometimes not sufficiently consulted prior to installation of new technology.

The technology is also seen as, to some extent, taking time away from relating directly to the patient, and there is a concern that the technology is potentially intrusive and liable to cause distress to patients. This view is not shared by the patients who generally see the technology as an essential part of their care and treatment. The patients have a high degree of confidence in the nurses and their ability to use the technology.

The availability of life sustaining technologies creates ethical dilemmas for nursing staff concerning the prolonging of 'low quality' life and decisions on priorities for the use of scarce resources. These dilemmas are an additional source of stress.

2.4   The Italian Study

The Italian Report includes case studies of technology in two very
different units - an Intensive Care Unit in a University Hospital and
a Hyperbaric Treatment Centre staffed mainly by volunteers.

2.4.1   The environments

The Intensive Care Unit studied is part of the University Hospital of
Padua.   The Unit, which can accommodate up to seven patients, has nine
qualified nurses and eight doctors.   The doctors are academics employed by
the University rather than the local health authority and alternate their
work between the Intensive Care Unit and anaesthetic duties in the
hospital's operating theatres.   A three shift system is operated with two
nurses and two doctors on duty for each shift.   The nurses shift cycle is
nine weeks.   The sequence is an afternoon, a morning, and a night shift on
consecutive days, followed by either a one-day or a two-day rest period.
Nursing duties comprise:

(1)   Assistance, supervision and cleaning of patients, and in particular
       the monitoring of vital functions.
(2)   Giving treatment.
(3)   Updating relevant parts of the patient's chart (this includes taking
       temperatures and pressures, and transcribing laboratory results).
(4)   Assisting the Unit's doctors and consultants during their
       examination of patients.
(5)   Checking visits by relatives, organsing their comings and goings and
       checking the timetable.

The patients are in seven beds around the perimeter of a single room.
There are no windows, and artificial lighting is on for 24 hours a day.   A
corner of the room contains a booth for a nurse to keep a check on patients
from a distance.   The corridor outside the room is used by relatives as a
waiting room and it contains a wall telephone.   Also off the corridor are a
room for the doctor on duty, a room for linen and equipment, and a small
kitchen.   Nursing staff generally use the doctors' room during their
breaks.

On average there are five patients in the Unit at a time and patients stay for an estimated duration of six days. The nurses on duty share responsibility for each patient. Nursing turnover is relatively high, on average nurses staying for two years. Absence due to illness is estimated at 8%.

The Hyperbaric Treatment Centre was founded in 1977 by the Padua Divers Club to treat specific disorders arising from underwater activity. In 1984 it began to treat patients sent by local health authority units from around the region. As a result a doctor from the Intensive Care Unit at Padua University Hospital has been seconded to coordinate and supervise all activities undertaken at the Centre.

The Centre is located in a building outside of the hospital and consists of a large room sub-divided into three areas - a waiting room, the working area containing a hyperbaric chamber, and a room for the doctor in charge.

A session lasts for about two hours and can accommodate up to two patients. A shift covers two successive sessions and normally involves three operators.

(a)   An operator at the console.
(b)   An operator going into the hyperbaric chamber with the patient.
(c)   An operator helping outside the chamber, for example, changing oxygen cylinders.

However there is not a strict demarcation of duties and staff also undertake associated duties such as assisting patients, checking and cleaning the chamber.

There are four shifts (eight sessions) worked a day involving 12 of the 27 operators attached to the Centre. The operators are all volunteers and all but four are male. They all hold underwater certificates and mostly work in non-hospital occupations. They have all undertaken a training course for hyperbaric chamber operators. There has been no turnover of operators during the first two years of activity and it is estimated that absence due to illness is 5%.

2.4.2 The technologies

In the Intensive Care Unit the technology in use can be divided into monitoring equipment and support equipment. An outline of the equipment available is provided in section 2.1. The set of equipment is available for each patient in the Unit though the individual patient alarms are not controlled by a central machine. Thus it is necessary for nursing staff to be able to observe all patients and equipment from a central point. The electronic monitoring technology was introduced into the Unit in 1982.

In the Hyperbaric Treatment Centre the main piece of equipment is the Hyperbaric chamber. This is a 4.3 metre long, 1.8 metre diameter steel cylinder. The space usable by patients is 2.1 metres in length and it can hold up to five people in a seated position. The chamber is able to create a pressure equivalent to 100 metre depth, although the average depth reached in treatment sessions is 18 metres. This is controlled from behind the cylinder at a vertical panel with pressure gauges for air and oxygen, and pressure regulators. Two dials in the middle of the panel show the barthymetric pressures which are gradually applied to the chamber's occupants.

The operator sits at a console and carries out compression and decompression operations according to plans laid out on special charts. The console operator can communicate with the occupants of the chamber through an intercom. The operator inside the chamber with the patients during the treatment session uses the intercom to report sphygomanometer pressure readings to staff outside. The inside of the chamber can be observed through a porthole.

2.4.3 The research methodology

In the Intensive Care Unit research methods involved the completion of established questionnaires by nursing staff and interviews with nurses, doctors, patients and their relatives.

(1)   The NIOSH questionnaire on work characteristics and job satisfaction
        was administered to 11 nurses associated with the unit.

(2) Yoshitake's 'F-scale' on physical and mental fatigue was also administered to 11 nurses. The F-scale comprise three sub-scales measuring (a) symptoms of sleepiness, (b) symptoms of difficulty in mental concentration, and (c) symptoms of physical discomfort associated with fatigue. Each nurse completed the questionnaire at the beginning and end of each of three consecutive shifts. In addition it was completed upon return to work after a two day rest period.

(3) The NIOSH 'Health Complaints' questionnaire on psychophysical symptoms of stress was administered to 11 nurses, who were asked to report the frequency with which a given symptom had occurred over the previous year.

(4) Interviews were carried out with two groups of four nurses. The aim was to investigate the nurses perceptions of stressors in their work, and in particular any problems connected with the use and maintenance of the equipment in the unit.

(5) Semi-structured interviews were conducted with a sample of former patients and their relatives. Criteria for selection were that during the previous three years the patient must have spent at least a week in the Unit in a conscious state. Post-traumatic patients were excluded from the sample. The selection procedure established a sample of 30 people, and whom 16 were traceable and agreed to be interviewed. Each ex-patient was invited to bring with them a relative who had been involved in their stay in the Unit. The focus of the interview was to investigate the experience of intensive care patients known as 'Intensive Care Syndrome' which concerns the display of psychological symptoms characterised by time and space disorientation and amnesia.

(6) A 'brainstorm' discussion group was held with four doctors to investigate their views on the nature and causes of 'Intensive Care Syndrome'.

Similar research methods were used in the Hyperbaric Treatment Centre. The NIOSH work characteristics and job satisfaction questionnaire, and the Health Complaints questionnaire were administered to ten operators.

Yoshitake's 'F-scale' was administered to ten operators at the beginning and end of a shift on the day before and the day after a rest break.

A group of four operators and the doctor associated with the Centre were interviewed to identify sources of stress and their importance. The work differences of being a volunteer at the Centre rather than an employee of the public health authority were also investigated.

2.4.4 The research findings

Job characteristics and stressors:

In the Intensive Care Unit eight of the eleven nurses reported they were fully satisfied with their work. However the work environmental stressors previously reported in the literature were also apparent in this Unit. The principal sources of stress were seen as:

(1) Being present at the death of patients, especially young ones, and witnessing therapeutic procedures which were intrusive and painful for patients.

(2) Being responsible for the monitoring of equipment which was liable to malfunction; in particular distinguishing between true and false alarms.

(3) Feeling inadequately trained to understand the functioning of the equipment, and thus unable to identify and rectify most frequently occurring malfunctions. Stress is seen as exacerbated by the frequent updating of equipment but with insufficient retraining, and by the turnover of staff.

(4) Experiencing difficulties in communicating with colleagues in the Unit. Prior to the introduction of the monitoring equipment, nurses checked the patient's condition directly at the bedside. In handing over to the next shift the main features of the patient's state of health were passed on from one nurse to another. This communication seemed to be a means of reducing anxiety about patients in danger. With the electronic monitoring technology vital functions are immediately monitored and do not need to be passed on. There is also uncertainty and therefore anxiety about the reliable functioning of the equipment.

(5)   Experiencing work overload, especially on the morning shift. This
        is because all planned (i.e. non emergency) admissions to the Unit
        take place during the morning because of hospital wide policy. The
        alternating shift system is used to spread this high morning
        overload across all nursing staff.

These stressors are off-set by a number of positive aspects of the work,
which is considered interesting and is seen as having precise aims and
clear lines of responsibility. Generally the level of cooperation between
staff is regarded as high.

In contrast, environmental factors in the Hyperbaric Treatment Centre are
rather different. Staff are mainly volunteers and have a high level of
motivation. They operate in a group free of hierarchical relationships or
highly structured tasks. The main stressors were seen as:

(1)   Problems of interacting with patients. Some patients have large
        skin lesions which emit unpleasant odours, others have serious
        illnesses such as multiple sclerosis and want advice from the
        operators on treatment. The operators, who have no nursing
        experience, have difficulties relating to these patients. In
        particular they experience anxiety about not being able to cope with
        clinical complications that might develop while the patient is in
        the hyperbaric chamber - even though the duty doctor is present in
        these circumstances. Operatives feel they have inadequate training
        in health care.

(2)   Work overload. The Centre attempts to meet all demands and this
        means sessions can go on until 2 am. Overload is also caused by
        patients and/or operators arriving late for sessions. Because
        operators feel a high degree of responsibility they are willing to
        work extra time even when this conflicts with their personal needs -
        this can cause anxiety and stress.

(3)   Relations with colleagues. Since there is no hierarchical structure
        problems that arise are seen as concerned with individual relation-
        ships rather than organisational structure.

(4)   Vigilance in monitoring the chamber. Because the pressure gauges
        have no sound alarms they must be kept under constant view. However
        in contrast to the Intensive Care Unit the equipment is seen as
        unproblematic to operate and is not a source of anxiety for staff.

Stress and fatigue experienced:

An analysis of the F-scale questions completed by nursing staff before and after shifts in the Intensive Care Unit gave the following results:

(1)   During their shifts on three consecutive days the nurses build up fatigue which is not eliminated during the eight hour break between shifts. The fatigue level at the beginning of a shift matches the level at the end of the previous shift.

(2)   The increase in the level of fatigue is most apparent in the 'sleepiness' sub-scale. The mental concentration and physical fatigue sub-scales are not significantly increased but show the same trend. However this trend is a matter for concern since a high degree of alertness is required at all times when nurses are on duty in Intensive Care.

(3)   The two-day break is sufficient to allow the normal level of functioning to return. This is probably due to the restoration of a normal rhythm of sleeping and waking.

An analysis of the psychophysical symptoms reported in the Health Complaints questionnaire produced an average score of 103 for the sample of intensive care nurses. This level of stress symptoms was not regarded as particularly high.

In the Hyperbaric Treatment Centre the principle findings from the F-scale were:

(1)   The shiftwork pattern in the Centre, which allows three to four days off between working days, means operators do not build up fatigue.

(2)   During the working day there is a reduction in the level of alertness but no fatigue effect with regard to mental concentration or physical fatigue.

The psychophysical symptoms reported in the Health Complaints questionnaire gave no indication of any significant work related complaints.

The impact of new technology on the nurses:

Although using and monitoring the new technology has become a major part of the job of the nurses in the Intensive Care Unit its use has not been included in the regulations contained in their duty manual. There are three aspects of the new technology which lead to stress for the nurses:

(1)   It can be difficult distinguishing whether an alarm is false or not.

(2)   Nursing staff have insufficient training in the use of the new technology. The problem is exacerbated because when staff have become familiar through on-the-job experience they are likely to transfer elsewhere. Nurses are aware of the possibility of making errors with the sophisticated equipment, but are reluctant to call the doctor unless it is really necessary. A unnecessary call is likely to be regarded as a sign of incompetence. Thus problems are generally solved by consulting a nurse with more experience of the equipment. This avoids calling the doctors who, in any case, are not seen as able to give particularly helpful advice on use of the equipment.

(3)   Use of the electronic equipment has resulted in a new type of patient care. Formerly the nurse checked the patient more frequently, because vital functions were not linked to a sound alarm system. The reduced checking of the patient's clinical condition has led to reduced communication of a patient's condition between nurses. Checking the vital functions also enabled nurses to talk to conscious patients and check their general condition. At present direct contact occurs less frequently.

The patients' view:

Of the 16 patients interviewed 14 said they could remember nothing of their stay in intensive care. This was despite having been selected because they had spent at least six days in the Unit and had been conscious at the time. The other two patients had difficulties recalling facts and specific episodes connected with their admission and the environment. Therefore the following findings draw heavily on the views of the patients' relatives:

(1)   All patients had been admitted to the Unit from another hospital ward and were returned there afterwards.

(2)   The main negative aspect of the time spent in the Unit was its short duration.

(3)   The co-operation between doctors and nurses was seen as a positive feature of the Unit.

(4)   Most (10 out of 14) relatives felt they had received sufficient information on the patient's condition at the time of admission.

(5)   There were mixed views about the physical environment of the Unit. Some regarded the continuous lighting and noise level preventing patients from resting; though 10 out of 14 thought the lighting levels were too low. The heating and ventilation were regarded as adequate although the room was also seen as full of unpleasant smells.

(6)   No information was provided to relatives or patients about the machines to which patients were linked.

(7)   The standard of assistance was judged better than expected by 12 out of 14 respondents.

Yet the lighting which is constantly on, the ever present noise, and the sight of other patients near death, induce a serious state of anxiety in the Unit. Doctors regard the best treatment for a conscious patient is to be discharged to another ward in the hospital.

'Intensive Care Syndrome':

The patients' experience in intensive care seems to have led to temporal-spatial disorientation and an almost total amnesia of the period of confinement in the Unit. This has been labelled 'intensive care syndrome' and a group discussion of doctors involved in intensive care was set up to try to establish its nature and cause. The following hypotheses were derived during the 'brainstorming' session:

(1)   Intensive care syndrome may arise because of the technologically advanced apparatus in use. This strongly held view cannot be generally sustained because patients in cardiac units are linked to equipment of comparable complexity, but do not exhibit the syndrome.

(2)   The technology in the Unit may influence the work organisation and structures which in turn bring about the syndrome, i.e. the beds are arranged so that they can be monitored and reached by a single nurse. This means the lights are continuously on for all patients

who can also observe the crises and deaths of other patients, and overhear discussions between staff. The constant lighting and lack of set routines in the Unit make it difficult for patients to differentiate time of day, and may lead to disorientation. This hypothesis views the experience as similar to that of a 'sensory deprivation' situation.

(3)   It can be further hypothesised that the invasive treatments administered in intensive care are causes of the syndrome. Some doctors view the main difference between a Cardiac Unit and Intensive Care Unit as not the technology but the invasive treatment in the latter. This hypothesis views the stress induced by invasive treatment and the real possibility of sudden deterioration as the cause of the syndrome. The doctors are aware that after a few days in Intensive Care conscious patients become disorientated and stressed, and tend to be increasingly unwilling to tolerate the monitoring terminals and emergency equipment. Some try to tear off breathing apparatus or humidifier, and to pull out needles. This reaction endangers patients' lives and thus doctors administer a massive sedation. This causes 'transient auterogade amnesia' which might explain the patients' memory gaps.

(4)   It can also be hypothesised that the syndrome is neurological in origin. It is possible that a patient with a cardio-vascular disorder has suffered transitory cerebral ischaemia which has characteristic symptoms of disorientation and memory failures.

Of these four possible explanations for 'intensive care syndrome' the first is unlikely, but the other three are plausible and merit further investigation.

2.4.5 Overview of the study

The Italian study has examined two quite different units, and although the stress experienced by staff in each is low there are substantially more stressors in the Intensive Care Unit. Some of these are characteristic of intensive care, such as dealing with serious ill or dying patients, and work overload. Fatigue accumulates between shifts for the nurses in intensive care and at the end of their third consecutive day their efficiency is probably reduced. There is no cumulation effect for the operators in the Hyperbaric Treatment Centre because they have substantial breaks between shifts. Stressors relating directly to new technology in intensive care focus around the nurses lack of confidence and competence in using the equipment. This is seen primarily as a training problem - more should be provided. The technology also has an indirect effect, in that it has led to a change in work organisation. There is reduced direct contact between nurses and patients and between nurse and nurse, particularly when changing over between shifts.

The reduced patient contact is perhaps particularly worrying because it appears that most, if not all, patients suffer from 'intensive care syndrome' if they have been conscious while in the Unit for 6 days or more. The causes of this syndrome - characterised by disorientation and amnesia - are not established, but may be due to:

(a)   A 'sensory deprivation' effect resulting from the physical environment.

(b)   Stress induced by invasive treatments and the anxiety of being surrounded by ill or dying patients. The sedation administered to relieve anxiety and rejection of the equipment may also cause amnesia.

(c)   Neurological impairment caused by transitory cerebral ischaemia.

The reduced patient contact, which is an indirect result of the new technology, leads to a reduction in opportunities to provide psychological support to the patients, and to explain the purpose of checks and treatments being carried out. It thus appears that although the new technology has been brought in to improve the curing function, it has resulted in a reduction in caring.

2.5   The UK Study

The UK Report comprises two studies. The first study examined the attitudes of student nurses to their work and to new technology, and assessed their level of general health. The second study was designed to examine the perceptions and attitudes of nurses who staff a new Intensive Care Unit, part of a new hospital planned to open during the course of the study. An aim was to investigate the effect on nurses of starting work with unfamiliar high technology equipment in a new unit. In the event the opening was delayed and the unit could not be included in the study. Thus only part one of the second study was completed – that is, the attitudes of intensive care nurses (who were transferring to the new unit) were assessed and were compared with the attitudes of a control group of nurses working in a medical coronary ward.

2.5.1   The environments

Study 1:

This study involved first and third year student nurses on the three year general training course at the University Hospital of Wales. The majority of the sample were training for State Registration, although a small number of the first year group were training for State Enrolment. The course involves theoretical teaching in the training institute and practical placements in the local hospitals. The following placements are included in the course:

Placement	Duration	Placement	Duration
Medical	8 weeks	Psychiatry	8 weeks
Surgical	24 weeks	Maternity/newborn	8 weeks
Geriatric	8 weeks	Paediatrics	8 weeks
Trauma	8 weeks	High dependency (ICU,	8 weeks
Theatre	8 weeks	CCU or cardio-thoracia)	

The study also involved nurses undertaking intensive care training. This course lasts for 30 weeks and in addition to 30 study days at the training school includes practical experience through the following placements:

Placement	Duration
10 bed cardiac/general ICU	8 weeks
4 bed general ICU	7 weeks
5 bed CCU	6 weeks
Anaesthetic department	1 week
Observation (any department)	1 week
Consolidation (catch up on any missed)	1 week

Study 2:

This study was intended to provide a more thorough investigation of the work situation in an Intensive Care Unit in the new hospital at Morriston, South Wales. Prior to the admission of patients to the new unit the staff had a familiarisation period which included an induction programme on how the Unit would function and on the use of the new equipment.

A 27 bed medical ward was also included in the study to provide a control group for the intensive care nurses. The ward functioned partly as the Coronary Care Unit for the hospital and therefore contained some sophisticated equipment - a cardiac monitoring system with central viewing room.

2.5.2 The technologies

No specific description of intensive care technologies is provided because the Intensive Care Unit to be studied did not open in time for the research to include it. However, the UK Report does provide in its Appendix C details of the technology to be used in the new unit. This includes:

(1) A description of the computer system for the Unit.
(2) The operation for the Engstrom Metabolic Computer.
(3) Design criteria for a Hewlett Packard Local Area Network in an Intensive Care Unit.

The appendix also contains an outline of the proposed induction programme for the new Unit and details of the Nursing Board's curriculum in General Intensive Care Nursing.

2.5.3 The research methodology

Prior to both studies contact was established with national and local officials in the National Health Service and with relevant Trade Unions. As a result of preliminary discussions and with an awareness of the severe time limitations on the study it was decided to:

(1)   Concentrate on the views and experience of nursing staff, particularly because of the ethical complications involved in working with patients.
(2)   Concentrate on intensive care.
(3)   Focus on student nurses.
(4)   Where possible use 'standard' scales and questionnaires for the assessment.

These considerations led to the design of two related studies.

Study 1:

This study had two parts, a questionnaire study involving student nurses and a small interview study involving nurses undergoing intensive care training. The same questionnaires were administered to both groups of nurses. These were: 'Computers in Hospitals' Attitude Scale (Hepworth and Fitter, 1982, 1982); General Health Questionnaire (Goldberg and Hillier, 1979); Minnesota Importance Questionnaire (Gay et al., 1971; Redfern, 1979).

The views of 41 first year students were compared with those of 42 third year students in order to investigate the effect of experience. The questionnaires were also administered to 10 nurses undertaking a 30 week intensive care training course.

Study 2:

The design for this study planned to assess the views of intensive care nurses:

(1)   Immediately prior to entering the new unit.
(2)   A month after the unit had opened.

(3)   Sometime later when they had become familiar with procedures and
        equipment.

Only phase (1) was able to be included in the study however. A control
group of nurses in a medical ward, which also functioned as a Coronary Care
Unit, was also included.

The sample of nurses included in the study was as follows:

	Intensive Care Unit	Medical/Coronary Ward (control)
Sisters	7	2
Staff Nurses	10	7
State Enrolled Nurses	11	–
Student Nurses	–	5
Night Staff	–	4
	28	18

The following questionnaires were administered to both groups of nurses:
'Computers in Hospitals' Attitude Scales (Hepworth and Fitter, 1981, 1982);
General Health Questionnaire (Goldberg and Hillier, 1979); 'Specific
Satisfactions' Job Satisfaction Scale (Hackman and Oldham, 1975); Social
Support Scales (Caplan et al., 1975; Moos, 1981); Depression Scales
(Karasek, 1979; Parkes, 1982); Job Content Scale (Quinn et al., 1979;
Karasek, 1979); Cognitive Failures Questionnaire (Broadbent et al., 1982).

2.5.4 The research findings

Study 1:

Analysis of the 'Computers in Hospitals' attitude scale revealed that first
year nursing students had a significantly more positive attitude towards
computers than did the third year students.

This difference may be a consequence of the training course, but may also
result from the greater amount of computer experience that the first years
had acquired (mainly through home computing or as a student prior to the
course). It was also found that the intensive care nurses had significantly

more positive attitudes to computers than the student nurses. This may reflect intensive care nurses' greater direct experience of technology.

The General Health Questionnaire (GHQ) scores were divided into 'high scorers' (those above a threshold which indicates the respondent is potentially diagnosable as psychiatrically ill) and 'low scorers'. High scorers were significantly more likely to disagree with the statement "computers have no place in anything so essentially human as medicine" (from the Computers in Hospitals scale). This may reflect a tendency to prefer communication with machines rather than communication with people. Generally high scorers on the GHQ had a more positive attitude to computers than did the low scorers.

Analysis of the Minnesota Importance Questionnaires revealed that third year students considered 'creativity', 'responsibility' and 'autonomy' to be more important in their ideal job than did first year students. Those who assigned greater importance to 'creativity' also had more negative attitudes to computers. Whereas those with more positive computer attitudes assigned greater importance to 'moral values'.

The following findings emerged from the interviews with the ten nurses at the end of their intensive care course:

(1)   Most of the nurses were specifically attracted to intensive care, mainly because of the opportunities for intensive (one-to-one) nursing. After the training half the nurses wanted a career in intensive care, the others did not want to specialise to that extent.

(2)   The most prominent difficulty experienced by the nurses was coping with the complex equipment, for example, "I was scared witless by it ... all the different drips and lines and all sorts of patients ... I don't think anything can prepare you for that". However, this problem was generally seen as solvable by adequate experience. A majority of nurses also perceived communications either with staff or patients to be a problem, and a source of stress. Communication with patients (verbal and non-verbal) was regarded as important even for unconscious patients. It was also seen as important to establish rapport with relatives and if necessary give them support. Several nurses also saw staff shortages as a major problem particularly the lack of experienced staff:

(3)   Of the 10 nurses, nine were enthusiastic about the training course, though five were critical of the preparation they were given for the use of intensive care technology. The main method of learning appeared to be on-the-job experience, though some of the nurses who provided advice did not appear to have a good enough knowledge of the technology to explain it adequately.

(4)   The design of the unit was important for five nurses. All the nurses favoured an open plan design that made it possible to see all beds from a single vantage point. One of the placement units was not liked because beds were in separate areas and this reduced the potential for communication between staff. Team work was seen as particularly important for intensive care staff. It is worth pointing out that the Italian study found adverse effects for patients which were attributed to the open-plan design. They were forced to all share the same environment and each others distress. It may be that there is a conflict between the ideal environment for nurses and for patients. The duration of the patients' stay in the unit was also seen as important. A short stay environment had the feel of a 'conveyor belt' and longer stay enabled nurses to get to know the patients.

(5)   Emergencies that develop in the unit were not seen as a source of stress, though breakdowns of equipment were. The monitor alarms were particularly criticised, because of the likelihood of false alarms. With some of the equipment it was difficult to discover the cause of the alarm. False alarms could be particularly stressful as one nurse reported: "Sometimes they do tend to sort of keep on alarming ... I think you probably need psychiatric help at the end of being on there - it's so loud, and it just keeps on alarming." There is a tendency to switch off the alarms if they continue to go off for no apparent reason; and then there is a danger that staff forget to turn them on again.

(6)   Five of the nurses said that, until they had become sufficiently familiar with the equipment, there was a tendency to concentrate on the equipment rather than the patient. As one nurse said,
"I'd only been there a month, but I was concerned with all the different charts and equipment. I was in a right panic and one of the senior staff said 'Now, just look at your patient, what does he look like, is he alright' ... since then I've always tried to remember that and it's something that you have to get used to."

'Machine caring' was viewed as part of the job of the intensive care nurse as well as the traditional patient caring. The former was a particular concern for inexperienced nurses.

Study 2:

Within the framework of the study completed to date, the views and attitudes of 22 nurses who transfered to the new Intensive Care Unit were compared with those of the 12 nurses in the medical ward control group.

The intensive care nurses had significantly more positive attitudes to computers than did the medical nurses. The intensive care nurses also reported significantly more somatic symptoms on the GHQ. They had also had more days off due to sickness in the previous month than had the medical nurses. These increased signs of illness could possibly be attributed to the recent move to a new job, rather than to the nature of the work itself. The intensive care nurses had a significantly higher level of depression as assessed by both depression scales.

However the medical nurses control group reported significantly greater time pressures than the intensive care nurses, though it should be recognised that the Intensive Care Unit had not opened to patients at the time of the assessment.

2.5.5 Overview of the study

It did not prove possible to investigate directly the experiences of nurses or patients in hospital units using new technology. Thus most of the findings derive from student nurses and from nurses undergoing training in intensive care.

New technology is seen as a problem and source of stress for nurses in Intensive Care Units, though these nurses also have a more positive attitude to the use of computers in health care. The problem is most acute when the nurses first work in intensive care. This appears to be a consequence of inadequate training in the use of complex equipment. At this point, in particular, nurses tend to see themselves as 'machine-carers' and find it difficult to focus on the patient.

Perhaps as a result of insufficient training, the nurses have difficulty using the monitoring technology and in particular identifying false alarms. This can be a source of stress leading to the switching off of the alarm mechanism.

Nurses in intensive care assign a higher level of importance to team work than other nurses and many prefer to work in an open-space environment where they can interact most readily with each other. This need may conflict with the need of patients for privacy and an environment which can be adjusted to their own individual needs.

2.6   The Netherlands Study

The Netherlands Report extends the scope of the project by making a
systematic comparison of work experiences of nursing in high and low
technology Units. Studies have been conducted in three Units in each of
two hospitals. The report places considerable emphasis on the organisation
of work in the Units studied and on the care provided to patients. It uses
quantitative techniques to examine the proportion of 'caring' and 'curing'
(technical) activities undertaken by nurses in each type of Unit. The
broader scope enables comparisons to be made of the effect of technological
complexity on the nurses' work and their experience of stress. It also
enables the researchers to investigate the hypothesis that, in the context
of a relatively 'fixed' health care budget, an indirect impact of high
technology health care is a 'draining' of resources from the lower
technology services.

By comparing Units in the two different hospitals the report enables an
assessment to be made of the effect of organisation and structure on
nurses' work.

2.6.1   The environments

Case studies were carried out in a large old University hospital (Groningen
Academic Hospital) and a medium sized hospital (Groningen Diakonessanhuis
Hospital). The University hospital has 1,105 beds and 2,180 nursing staff
(1,240 full-time equivalents). It also has a teaching and research role.
The Diakonessenhuis Hospital, which is a private, non-profit enterprise,
has 422 beds and 390 nursing staff (362 full-time equivalents). The
organisation structure of the Diakonessenhuis Hospital is much less complex
than the University hospital. The latter has a significant degree of
bureaucracy, with decision making following strictly hierarchical lines.
However, it is often unclear to people working in the various departments
where and how decisions are made, where information can be obtained, and
how decisions can be influenced. The power structure at the
Diakonessenhuis, on the other hand, is much more transparent - the lines of
command are shorter and less rigid. A conscious attempt is made to conduct
a flexible, practical policy, and to avoid bureaucracy as much as possible.

The University hospital being larger and covering a larger catchment area also offers more specialised services. A consequence of this is that the University nurses are more likely to be involved in specialised work. Due to the limited size of the Diakonessenhuis Hospital, promotion is, in practice, only possible if a nurse takes a special training course, such as in Cardiac Care. Career prospects are linked to technically oriented training, but this training is only available if the hospital needs nurses to have extra qualifications. The shift work system makes it practically impossible for nurses to take a course in their own time. The nurses in the University Hospital are in government service and are paid more than the privately employed Diakonessenhuis nurses. The jobs and terms of employment of the latter depend directly on the efficiency of their business organisation.

The high technology unit studied in the University hospital was the Intensive Care Unit, and the lower technology units were the Paediatrics Unit and the Surgical Unit.

The Intensive Care Unit accommodates up to 16 patients (bed occupancy is 83%) some of whom are in single rooms and some in rooms with up to eight beds. They are usually admitted following major surgery or when critically ill. The average duration of stay is 3.15 days. About 80 nurses work in the Unit (16 part-time), of whom about 45% are male. Nurses remain in the Unit for three to four years on average, so although it takes about a year to become familiar with the work and the technology there are many experienced nurses in the Unit. Absence through illness is low (6.5%). Work is carried out on an overlapping four-shift system. There are at least 13 nurses on duty at any time. If possible nurses work for two or three days with the same patient and each nurse is assigned to one or two patients per duty.

The Paediatrics Unit has 39 beds, made up of two and four bed rooms and three single rooms. Within it there is a medium care unit and a babies ward. Patients in the medium care unit are watched continually with the aid of monitors. The Unit caters for general and orthopaedic surgical cases and cases of trauma, oncological, urological, cardiac and respiratory disorders. The duration of stay for patients varies from three days to four to six weeks. There is a nursing staff of 35 (13 part-time), and it takes about six months for staff to become familiar with the work and to be able to work on their own in the medium care unit. The nurses work in one of four teams, each responsible for its own section. During the day two nurses work together in each section. In medium care there are always two nurses with the patients.

The Surgical Unit has 32 beds in two large wards. There is little privacy since the wards also function as passageways for visitors and staff. The Unit has cases of trauma, orthopaedics and vascular disorders. Nearly all patients are conscious but are confined to bed and need considerable basic care. They remain in the Unit from four to five days to six weeks. There are 21 nursing staff and turnover is relatively high (average two year stay), since the workload is heavy and many nurses want to gain experience elsewhere. Nurses are assigned to a group of six patients and carry out all duties except medical procedures (only sisters are authorised to carry out certain medical procedures such as intravenous injections).

The high technology unit studied in the Diakonessenhuis Hospital was the Cardiology Unit, and the lower technology units were the Neurology Unit, and the Internal Medicine Unit.

The Cardiology Unit has eight beds with central monitoring facilities for acute cases and two follow-up units of 12 and 7 beds respectively. Two thirds of the patients are admitted with acute heart conditions, and most are fully conscious. The average duration of stay is from seven to ten days, four days of which are spent in Cardiac Care. Nineteen nurses work in the Unit (six part-time), 13 of whom are Cardiac Care nurses. Approximately half the nurses are male. There are five nurses and student nurses on day duty and three in the evenings and at night, at least two of whom are qualified Cardiac Care nurses. Staff turnover is fairly high, if nurses can find suitable alternatives, because of the strain and tension in the Unit. Eight nurses were reported as leaving within three months, mainly to go to the ICU at the University Hospital where pay was higher and more varied in cases were available. However the nursing management is seen as supportive and all registered nurses take it in turns to function as the senior nurse in each of the three sections. Each section has a team of nurses who do their own planning, allocating and carrying out of duties. There is a good deal of contact with patients who want information about their condition. There is also much involvement with patients' relatives, and for some critical cases relatives are allowed to stay overnight in the unit. However there is no separate area for relatives or for discussions and meetings with relatives or amongst staff. Thus the accommodation is seen as inadequate for staff, for patients and for relatives. A particular feature of the Cardiology Unit is that two-thirds of patients are acute admissions who arrive unpredictably (12 acute cases per week on average). They require immediate and substantial attention and if they arrive on the evening or night shift no doctors are present. Nurses thus have to carry out unauthorised duties (medical procedures such as setting up and attaching drips). The consequence of emergencies is regular but unpredictable pressures with excessive work needing to be carried out in insufficient time. In particular, if when an emergency arrives all the Cardiac Care beds are occupied a patient must be 'decanted' to the follow-up section, thereby disturbing other patients who are seriously ill.

The Neurology Unit accommodates 25 neurological, six ear, noise and throat (ENT), and six internal medicine patients. The Unit is divided into three sub-units with six, three and two bedded rooms and a number of single rooms. The majority of neurological patients are seriously ill and cannot be communicated with. They often stay in the Unit for a long period, and a good deal of basic care is needed, involving heavy physical work. ENT patients usually only remain a few days. There are 17 nursing staff (four part-time), and turnover is relatively low, but has increased when opportunities to transfer arose in the recent past. During the day nurses is allocated to each of the three sub-units. In the evening and night two nurses are on duty in the Unit.

The Internal Medicine Unit accommodates 33 internal patients and two dermatological patients (bed occupancy is 57%). Patients usually stay for from two to three weeks, occasionally up to three months. Some patients can do a lot for themselves, others need a lot of care. The Unit has 13 nurses (four part-time) and nine student nurses. There has been a fairly high turnover for several years due to problems which have been resolved. The turnover is now substantially lower. Nurses have close contact with patients, particularly those that spend a long time in the Unit, but there is a distance between doctors and nurses, attributed to a lack of consultation.

2.6.2 The technologies

Only the Intensive Care Unit at the University Hospital and the Cardiac
Care Unit at the Diakonessenhuis Hospital use high level technology.
Therefore the description of equipment characterics is restricted to these
two units, and details may be found in the Netherlands Report (Part III,
chapter 2.3).

Patients in the Intensive Care Unit are constantly monitored and their
bodily functions regulated. Each bed is surrounded by a large amount of
equipment and each patient is watched, checked and attended 24 hours a day.
The Cardiac Care Unit also has a high level of instrumentation but it is
mainly used for monitoring and regulating cardiac function and patients are
not usually suffering from any other illness or surgical wounds. The Unit
is made up of a number of connected rooms and monitoring takes place at a
central point where the monitors are installed. The Intensive Care Unit
requires more nurses per patient than the Cardiac Care Unit because of the
large number of machines and the individual monitoring that each patient
requires. Because of the many acute cases in the Cardiac Care Unit and the
lower availability of doctors, nurses need to exercise greater initiative
in the use of equipment and medication, and therefore carry a heavy burden
of responsibility.

In the Surgical, Neurological and Internal Medicine Units a very limited
amount of equipment is available - mainly restricted to oxygen and infusion
apparatus and suction pumps. Paediatrics is the only Unit with a Medium
Care Unit using monitoring equipment. Apart from this Paediatrics has
little instrumentation.

2.6.3 The research methodology

The study was in three parts. In the first, national developments in
patient care and the nursing profession were assessed. Against this background the introduction of new technology was considered. Evidence was
provided by representatives of employers and unions in the health service
and by the public authorities concerned.

The second part of the study assessed the organisation of patient care in two hospitals, based on structured interviews with management, administrative staff, departmental heads and representatives of the nursing staff in the six units studied. In addition observations were made and hospital records studied.

The third part of the study was a questionnaire survey of nurses views on the impact of new technology on the content and performance of their jobs. Questionnaires were administered to all members of the nursing staff in each of the six units over a two-week period. The average response rate was 78%, with very little variation between Units. The sample of nurses surveyed was as follows:

Hospital	High technology	Low technology
University	Intensive Care Unit n = 76	General Surgery Unit n = 21
		Paediatrics Unit n = 23
Diakonessenhuis	Cardiology Unit n = 16	Neurology Unit n = 14
	Cardiac Care Unit n = 7	Int Medicine Unit n = 13

The research design allowed a comparison to be made of the differences between the high and low technology units, and between the units in the two hospitals.

The questionnaires were used to assess the impact of technology and hospital organisation on the following:

(1)   The proportion of 'curing' and 'caring' activities in the nurses' work: a 160 item list of work activities, grouped into 36 categories, was drawn up with the help of nursing staff and each item was assessed for its degree of caring and degree of curing.

(2)   The actual job content: the nurses' actual work tasks were assessed
        according to the above 36 categories so that the proportion of
        'caring' and 'curing' activities could be determined. A question-
        naire (Overton et al., 1977) was used to assess variety of nursing
        tasks and the 'Organisation Stress' questionnaire (Reiche et al.,
        1979) was used to assess level of autonomy and scope for initiative.

(3)   The preferred job content: Nurses were asked to say how long they
        would prefer to spend on each work task so that the profile of
        preferred 'caring' and 'curing' activities could be determined.

(4)   The potential conflict between preferred and actual job content:
        the preferred and actual times were compared for the 36 categories
        of work tasks, and a difference (or conflict) score calculated.

(5)   The presence of stress: This was assessed using standard question-
        naires. (i) Psychosomatic complaints (the VOEG State of Health
        Questionnaire; Dirken, 1967); (ii) Stress experienced and the need
        for treatment (Meijman et al., 1984); (iii) 'Reluctance to work'
        and 'How important is my job?' (Meijman et al., 1984).

(6)   The relationship between the presence of job conflicts (4 above) and
        stress (5 above).

2.6.4   The research findings

The primary aim of the Netherlands study was to examine the effects of new
technology as revealed by the differences between the high and low level
technology units. This section focuses on the differences found though,
unless stated otherwise, the findings are also consistent with the job
characteristics, stressors and experienced stress in the high technology
units described in the previous sections of this report.

Job characteristics and stressors:

The physical working conditions in the high technology units (ICU and CCU)
were inferior to those in the low technology units, in particular due to
excessive noise levels, poor ventilation and dry air. Although there were
no significant differences between the ICU and CCU, overall the physical
conditions in the University Hospital were inferior to those in the
Diakonessenhuis Hospital.

The 'Organisational Stress' questionnaire indicated that many nurses in all the Units 'sometimes or frequently' experienced stress due to constant time pressures. But the nurses in the low technology units reported significantly more stress due to time pressure. Also there is significantly more time pressure stress in the CCU than the ICU, as might be expected from the high number of acute admissions. This questionnaire also indicated that rarely do nurses have to carry out duties which conflict with other work which needs to be done. Incidents were particularly low in the ICU.

Uncertainty factors in the nurses' work were assessed with the Overton questionnaire. Significantly greater uncertainty was found in the high technology units. This is due to more complex problems and treatments, and greater patient dependence on intervention and the quality of nursing. Treatment in the high technology units is primarily geared to altering the patient's condition by means of technical equipment. In the low technology units a gradual recovery process takes place, without the need for frequent intervention. Thus the high technology units seem to require more patient and situation specific responses from the nursing staff.

However, nurses in the high technology units have less job variety because they deal with a more homogeneous group of patients, and therefore a narrower range of procedures are used. Possibly for this reason, high technology nurses experience more monotony in their work and spend much of their time on technical nursing activities. In intensive care, in particular, observing the machine monitors is monotonous. The high technology nurses also reported significantly more difficulty staying awake at night.

The extent of 'autonomy in planning and organising work' (Karasek, 1979) did not differ significantly between nurses in high and low technology units. However the low technology nurses had significantly more 'autonomy in policy-making with respect to the unit and patient care'. Consistently, the high technology nurses had significantly fewer opportunities for participation with superiors in decision-making. Both groups of nurses reported receiving little support from superiors or colleagues in their work.

The proportion of caring and curing (technical) activities:

The study has classified all nursing activities according to their curing (technical) and caring components. The technical aspect is defined as the use of a nursing technique, e.g. the use of equipment, physiotherapy treatment, or even the application of an interview technique. Technical procedures deal primarily with the diseased organism or the disease itself. The caring aspect is defined as looking at the basic needs of the patient (washing the patient, changing bed linen etc.), and the psychosocial care of the patient (giving reassurance or advice etc.). Caring activities thus include procedures for basic care, and psychosocial guidance of the patient as an individual.

To assess the relative proportions of caring and curing components in nursing work, 164 nurses (from the six units) were asked to use the above definitions to rate the degree of caring and curing in each of the 160 nursing activities on a 5-point scale for each dimension. The nurses were also asked to estimate how much of their own daily work consisted of caring and how much of curing.

The results were presented on a two dimensional graph (caring/curing) and indicated that the 36 categories of nursing activity were grouped into five major clusters. These clusters appeared robust in that very similar groupings emerged for the high and low technology units, and for the University and Diakonessenhuis Hospitals. One difference that did emerge was that the nurses in the low technology units tended to give all the activities a slightly higher 'caring' score, perhaps indicating a greater orientation towards 'caring'. The five clusters (A to E) are listed in table 2.6.1, along with the 36 categories of activities that they comprise.

Table 2.6.1:

The five clusters which resulted from the assessment by 164 nurses of
36 categories of nursing activity (caring and curing components)

Cluster A:

Psycho-social care:
- providing information and guidance to patients and their relatives
- encouraging patients to get up, cough up, eat, drink
- helping patients to move, cough, eat, drink
- occupational therapy
- preparing patients for examination or treatment

Basic physical care:
- washing etc. of patients
- laying out deceased patients
- answering bells (various 'in between' jobs)

Cluster B:

Simple technical procedures:
- keeping lists
- work involved in checking the primary bodily functions
- simple procedures required for making diagnoses
- simple procedures involved in giving transfusions (by drip)
- procedures involving stomach tubes
- preparatory work

Complex technical procedures:
- procedures for attaching patients to monitors
- controlling and monitoring other than basic bodily functions
- complex procedures required for making diagnoses (ECG's etc.)
- complex procedures involved in giving transfusions and intravenous
  injections
- procedures involving the patient's respiration

cont'd ...

Table 2.6.1 cont'd ...

Cluster C:

Combined caring/curing procedures:
- observing and assessing the patient's condition
- the dressing and treatment of wounds
- the patient's medication (other than by transfusion)
- duties connected with the risk of bedsores etc.
- assisting the doctor in examining and treating patients
- procedures connected with intestinal feeding
- procedures connected with evacuation
- procedures adopted in acute or critical situations
- procedures connected with the function of the lungs

Cluster D:

Domestic work:
- domestic tasks, serving tea, coffee and meals
- cleaning work, sluice-room

Cluster E:

Organisational activities:
- writing reports
- helping and instructing new nurses
- teaching activities
- consultations and verbal reports
- patient-oriented policy, organisational and planning activities
- unit-orientated policy, organisational and planning activities

The magnitude of caring and curing components for each of the five clusters is as follows:

	Cluster	Caring Component	Curing Component
A	Psycho-social care and Basic physical care	High	Low
B	Simple and complex technical procedures	Low	High
C	Combined caring/curing procedures	High	High
D	Domestic work	Low	Low
E	Organisational activities	Moderate	Moderate

The nurses' estimates of the proportion of caring and curing activities in their work revealed that the nurses in the high technology units carried out many more curing activities, and that nurses in low technology units carried out many more caring activities. However there were no significant differences betwen the proportions of caring and curing in the two hospitals.

Nurses' actual and preferred job profiles:

The nurses were asked to estimate how much time they spent on each of the 36 categories of activity (table 2.6.1), using a 7 point scale (0 = 'no time at all'; 6 = 'more than 2.5 hours per day'). The nurses were also asked to assess the amount of time they preferred to spend on each activity using the same 7 point scale, and bearing in mind the circumstances in their Unit and their own abilities. The results, shown in table 2.6.2, indicate that much time is spent on simple technical procedures, especially in the high technology units. These units also spend much of their time on complex technical procedures, whereas the low technology units spend very little time on these activities. Whereas the high technology nurses are satisfied with this emphasis on complex procedures, they would prefer less time on simple technical procedures. The low technology nurses would like to spend more time on complex procedures. The high technology nurses also spend more time on combined caring/curing procedures, though both groups are satisfied with the amount of time they devote to these activities.

Table 2.6.2:
Results of the survey to determine the actual and preferred job profile, broken down into types of unit and hospital (average scores of amount of time on the activity: 0 = none; 6 = > 2.5 hours)

Type of activity	Total Group (n = 164)	Level of technology		Type of hospital	
		High	Low	University (ICU)	Diakonessenhuis (CCU)
Psychosocial care					
current situation	2.87	2.49	3.37	2.46	2.51
preferred situation	3.22	2.84	3.73	2.74	3.23
Basic physical care					
current situation	2.67	2.35	3.11	2.26	2.86
preferred situation	2.42	2.17	2.77	2.17	1.76
Simple technical procedures					
current situation	3.06	3.41	2.65	3.61	2.78
preferred situation	2.90	3.15	2.61	3.32	2.55
Complex technical procedures					
current situation	2.21	3.42	0.69	3.84	2.40
preferred situation	2.40	3.31	1.20	3.69	2.34
Combined caring/curing					
current situation	2.72	2.91	2.51	3.06	2.32
preferred situation	2.82	2.97	2.67	3.11	2.41
Domestic duties					
current situation	2.10	1.69	2.63	1.36	3.07
preferred situation	1.30	1.13	1.52	1.19	0.64
Organisational activities					
current situation	1.84	1.52	2.25	1.37	2.62
preferred situation	2.73	2.64	2.86	2.53	3.25

The low technology nurses spend considerably more time on psycho-social care and basic physical care than the high technology nurses. However, both groups would like to spend less time on basic physical care and more time on psychosocial care. This difference between preferred and actual time on psychosocial care is particularly strong for the nurses in the Cardiac Care Unit.

Domestic duties are unpopular with all the groups of nurses, though nurses have to do more in the low technology units. The Cardiac Care Unit is an exception in that nurses report spending most of their time on these duties and would prefer to spend least. The low technology nurses spend more time on organisational activities, though all the groups would prefer to spend more time. This reflects a desire to be more involved with policy-making and organising and planning for their unit.

Overall there is a desire to be more involved in responsible and complex activities, and less tied up with routine tasks such as domestic work.

Stress experienced:

The Netherlands study used standard questionnaires to examine four possible types of stress reaction. These are summarised in table 2.6.3.

Table 2.6.3:
Results of a survey of stress reactions, broken down into types of unit and hospital (average scores, higher indicates more stress)

Unit/Hospital	Psychosomatic illness	Need for recuperation	Reluctance to work	Feeling overworked
High technology	3.4	4.0	1.2	2.0
Low technology	3.6	4.3	2.0	2.4
University	3.2	3.8	1.4	2.0
Diakonessenhuis	4.2	4.8	2.1	2.8

Each of the stress measures produced similar results. Nurses in the Diakonessenhuis hospital found their work more stressful. This confirmed the impression gained from the interviews and observations in the two hospitals that the workload in the Diakonessenhuis was heavier as a result of lower staffing levels. There was also a small, but non-significant, tendency for the nurses in the low technology units to experience more stress in their work.

An assessment was made of the relationship between reported stress and job conflict, as measured by the discrepancy between actual and preferred job profiles. No relationship was found for the nurses in the high technology units. However there was a link for the nurses in the low technology units who had reported more job conflicts. The stress seems to be attributable to the desire for a reduction in domestic work and physical caring, and an increase in complex technical activities.

Training and the use of new technology:

Working with new technology requires training orientated towards the technical side of health care. However it is difficult for training programmes to keep pace with the rate at which the technology is developing. This has led to situations in which new technology is introduced without sufficient training of the staff who must operate it. Training given by the suppliers has not solved the problem because many of the difficulties have arisen after installation, when the equipment is in use.

Nursing work in the high technology units has required extra training, and this has been rewarded by an increased salary. In the context of poor promotion prospects for nurses, working with new technology is therefore seen as an opportunity for promotion, and a career in nursing in the Netherlands is linked to some form of technological training. This may, in part, explain why a relatively large proportion of male nurses work in high technology units (50% male as compared with 5-15% in low technology units).

The concentration of funds and training opportunities in the high technology units is reported as reducing the opportunities for nurses in the low technology units to advance. Although the development of medical knowledge and methods of treatment makes it desirable that nurses in these units receive extra training, there are few opportunities available, and nurses are generally unable to take courses in their own time because of the shift work.

There is evidence to suggest that the introduction of new technology does not relieve the workload for nursing staff, and may even increase it - despite the claims of suppliers. For example, computer monitoring equipment was installed in the Cardiac Care Unit five years ago. It was expected to save time and personnel because it would be no longer necessary to walk up and down the ward to observe the monitors and the patients. The computer would also interpret the various warning signals at the different alarm levels. In practice, although the production of different alarm levels reduced stress, the computer made much more data available and this required complex interpretation. Thus the time saved in moving about was offset by the increased time spent on the more complex and intensive monitoring.

Similarly the introduction of a Haemodynamic monitor enabled a constant measurement of blood pressure in the heart by means of a tiny tube inserted via an artery. However the equipment necessitated extra patient care, since patients were immobilised and it was difficult to keep the insertion wound sterile. Errors of measurement occurred regularly and required difficult decisions on whether to call the cardiologist. The patient was often uneasy about the monitoring and required additional psychological care.

Both these examples show that the introduction of new technology can result in no change or an increase in the intensity of work provided by nursing staff. This general picture is in contrast to the popular view of the impact of new technology in many branches of industry and commerce, where it is believed that substantial savings in staff time can be achieved.

The effect on the patient:

There have been few reported problems with the quality or reliability of the equipment used in the units studied. It seems that the standard of observation, diagnosis and treatment is improved with the aid of technology. However, some specific problems for the patients have been identified.

(1)   The availability of more tests or diagnostic procedures makes it likely that they will be used, even if not strictly necessary.

(2)   The technical procedures often require more dressing of wounds, involving a greater risk of infection. The patients are also more immobilised, with associated risks of thrombosis, bedsores etc.

(3)   There is increased dependence on the machines which monitor and provide support functions. This may induce anxiety in patients, particularly if they haven't been sufficiently informed about the procedures.

(4)   There is increased focus on the patient's non-functioning part or symptom. The patient is more likely to be reduced to an object with a particular problem which can be treated by technical intervention.

2.6.5 Overview of the study

The Netherlands study has examined six units in two hospitals. It has focused on the level of technology in use and the type of hospital as predictors of the characteristics of nursing work and the type of patient care provided.

One of the main conclusions is that the impact of new technology is not confined to the high technology units where it is mainly found. There is an indirect effect whereby additional resources are provided for high technology units at the expense of other units. This 'draining' effect is a consequence of technological expansion in a climate of relatively fixed overall health care budgets.

The use of advanced technology has a substantial effect on the content of nursing work. The increased need for technical procedures ('curing' activities) means there is less time for other activities. There appears to be a hierarchy of activities with those at the top demanding and getting most time spent on them, and those of the bottom being relatively starved as a consequence. This hierarchy is:

(1)   Technical nursing.
(2)   Basic physical care and domestic duties.
(3)   Psychosocial care.
(4)   Organisational activities.

Thus in high technology units there is a higher proportion of curing (technical) activities and correspondingly less caring (psychosocial) activities. Domestic duties, although rated as low on both curing and caring components are a necessity and therefore take priority over most other activities. In contrast, organisational activities, which are also not related directly to curing or caring, have lowest priority. However these latter activities include the planning and organising necessary if nurses are to feel effective at their work. Lack of time for these activities can be particularly stressful for nurses since they cannot participate in decision making or feel in control of their environment. However, the evidence from the case studies indicates this is more a consequence of general lack of nursing resources rather than the use of technology per se. The shift in the proportion of 'curing' activities at the expense of 'caring' activities does seem to be a direct consequence of the introduction of new technology.

There is no evidence that the nurses in the high technology units experience more stress than those in the low technology units, though the nurses in the Diakonessenhuis Hospital, where the staffing levels are lower, report more stress than in the other hospital.

2.7 Ward Based Management Information Systems

With the exception of Intensive Care Units, computerised information processing systems have as yet had no major impact on nursing work. Nor have the information systems been very apparent to patients in the ordinary hospital ward. This is because, to date, these systems have supported functions peripheral to the nursing process itself. Yet there is evidence to suggest that management information systems will develop in hospitals, and as they become more ward based they will begin to affect the core of the nursing process - the basic tasks frequently performed by nurses under considerable physical and psychological pressure. Whether these developments will lead to an improvement in the nurses' and patients' environment remains to be seen.

In hospitals computer systems were first applied for general administration - accounts, wages, patients' invoices and financial statistics. More recently computer systems have been introduced into laboratory data processing and pharmacy management (Reichertz and Lordieck, 1984). Administrative systems have also been introduced into the hospital stores and out-patient departments.

There has been much discussion of the potential of integrated hospital information systems (HIS) which can co-ordinate the various administrative, medical, nursing and technical departments. However such systems only exist as developmental systems in a few large hospitals. Within this framework of developments the nursing sector is just beginning to come into contact with computer based information systems, though the extent of contact would not generally warrant the description 'computerised nursing processes'.

A schematic outline of computer based information systems relevant to nursing is provided in figure 2.7.1. Two broad functions can be distinguished. Firstly, there are 'external' communication functions, concerned with information flows between wards and external units such as the pharmacy, laboratory, stores, service departments, kitchen, admissions etc. Secondly, there are internal ward services, concerned mainly with the support and control of nursing administration within the ward, for example, planning, records, nursing requirements, recruitment, duty rostering and time keeping.

82

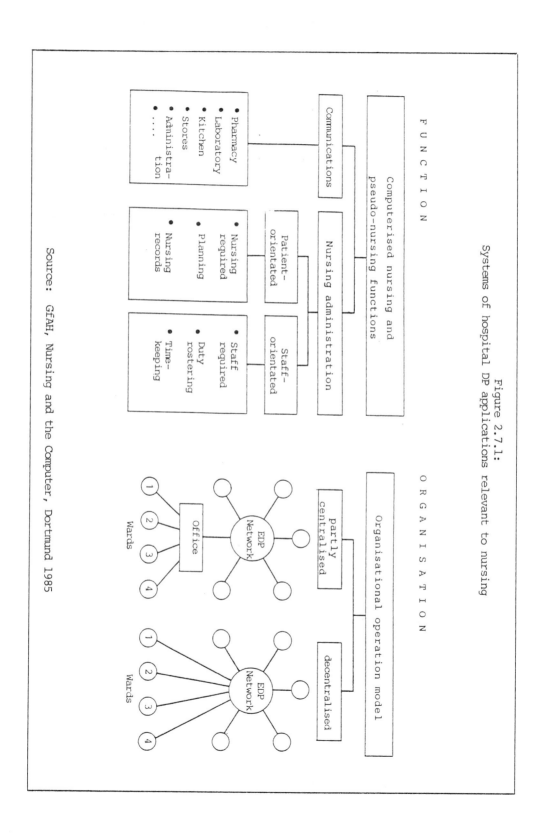

Figure 2.7.1:
Systems of hospital DP applications relevant to nursing

Source: GfAH, Nursing and the Computer, Dortmund 1985

These functions can be based on two quite distinct organisational models:

(a)   Partly centralised. A special organisational unit is set up between the nurses and the hospital information systems connecting with the other departments. Such a unit can service a group of wards, is staffed by a specialist (usually non-nursing) secretary, and is equipped with appropriate computer terminals.

(b)   Decentralised. Each ward has its own terminals operated by nursing staff, and is directly connected to the hospital information system.

Hospital information system designers have a choice as to which alternative to pursue. Each has its own financial and organisational implications - and also will be likely to have an impact on the nature and quality of nursing work.

2.8   The Federal Republic of Germany Study

The German Study addresses itself to the impact of ward based information systems on nurses' work. Partially centralised systems, emphasising communication functions (see section 2.7) are more commonly found in German hospitals, and one of these is the subject of the case study. However the report also consider the implications of decentralised systems in contrast to partially centralised ones, and uses its conclusions to put forward recommendations for the future development of ward based management information systems.

2.8.1   The environment

The case study was carried out in a teaching hospital with 1,473 beds and 4,398 staff, of whom 964 are nurses. The average bed occupany is 82%, and the average duration of patient stay is 10.8 days. There is a general belief amongst the nursing staff that there is a chronic shortage of staff in the hospital. This view was reinforced by a recent economic analysis by external consultants which was unable to recommend any rationalisations resulting in staff savings.

Support services to the wards are provided from central locations. These include domestic and catering services, paramedical services and therapy. This clustering of services has created the conditions necessary for the implementation of information technology. The centralisation has resulted in a high traffic flow of patients, goods and information between the service sectors and the hospital wards. These have received major rationalisations. Goods containers (for transporting food, laundry, refuse etc.) are conveyed by a computer controlled system and a separate small conveyor is used for patients' files, X-rays, laboratory samples and results etc. This rationalising of information exchange has facilitated the development of the computer network which has been installed (see section 2.8.2).

The case study itself was carried out in two selected nursing departments, comprising three urological wards and five internal medicine wards. Each department has four wards, four staff duty rooms, a supply depot, and the departmental office. The office is staffed by a departmental secretary who uses the computer terminal for communicating with the Hospital Information System. The office is also linked to the small conveyor network. The supply depot is the point of transfer for arriving and departing goods containers as well as an intermediate store for nursing supplies. One consequence of the complete rationalisation of the transport system is that nursing staff can remain in their ward during working hours. It is, as a rule, unnecessary for them to leave the ward. The wards, of course, operate for 24 hours a day on a three shift system, though the office is only staffed Monday to Friday, 6.30 am to 5 pm. Access to the computer is only available during these periods.

Each department has 20 beds in single and two-bed rooms, and is staffed by eight nurses (full-time equivalents). Nursing turnover is very low and absence due to illness is 8% for the urology wards, and 5.5% for the medical wards.

2.8.2 The information system

The linking of the wards to the computerised Hospital Information System via the departmental offices is an example of a partially centralised system (section 2.7). An outline of the network in operation in the hospital is provided in figure 2.8.1. Its operation is described by chronicling its use during a patient's typical stay in the hospital.

During the first few days in hospital numerous diagnostic and therapeutic procedures are carried out. These generate an intensive flow of information between the ward and external services. A large proportion of these requests were transmitted by the computer system to the departments concerned. A request is initiated by someone, usually the ward sister, filling in a special input form. Patient identification details are put on the form with a computer printed self-adhesive label based on the admissions details. This has simplified the form filling work (but not eliminated it). The completed forms and relevant enclosures (blood or urine samples etc.) are taken to the departmental office. The secretary enters the data into the terminal and sends off the samples via the small conveyor system.

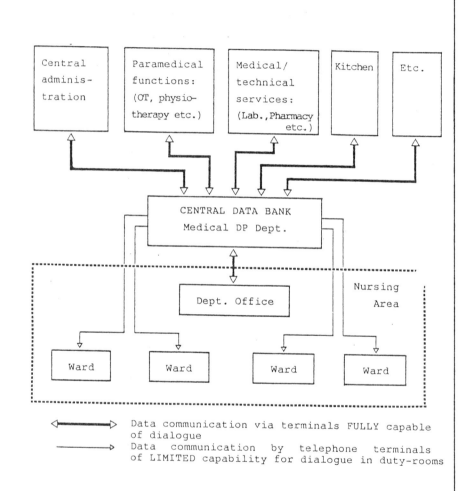

Figure 2.8.1:

Data processing network at the hospital researched
in the case study

Source: GfAH, Nursing and the Computer, Dortmund 1985

The return flow of goods or services requested is mainly directed back via the departmental office or supply depot. However the results of laboratory tests are sent directly to the ward. Each ward duty room is linked to the central computer by a telephone link and a micro-printer. The results are sent direct to the printer which acts as a telex machine. The printout is on a self-adhesive label which may be stuck to the patient's file.

The duty room terminal can also be used to request laboratory data. Numeric codes (the nurses' password and the patient's number) are entered on the telephone terminal, and a programmed key is pressed to indicate which information is required. Other programmed keys on the terminal permit the retrieval of information on the number of beds, and on medication ordered for the ward.

The patient is discharged by the doctor in charge. The ward sister completes a form and the data is entered into the computer by the departmental secretary.

Thus the main function of the Hospital Information System is to permit information transfers between wards and external services. There is no computerisation related directly to nursing functions, for example, duty rosters, nursing planning or nursing records. The major part of computer communications is carried out by the secretary on the departmental office terminal. Not even in exceptional circumstances is this terminal used by nursing staff. Thus ward staff have very little direct access to the hospital network. The hardware in the duty rooms is practically incapable of dialogue – it is essentially for data output only. Data input is achieved by filling in the appropriate form for transmission by the secretary.

2.8.3 The research methodology

The study was based on qualitative research methods. Detailed, semi-structured individual and group interviews were conducted, and observations were made of work processes, primarily in the departmental offices.

Individual interviews were conducted with the secretaries in each of the two departmental offices. Individual and group interviews took place with ward management, sisters and nurses. Supplementary discussions took place with experts in central nursing management and with the nursing services manager of a specialist clinic.

All the investigations had the prior agreement of the hospital management (in particular the nursing services management).

2.8.4 The research findings

The use of the new technology and its effect on job content:

The Hospital Information System does not directly support the nurses in the execution of their duties. In the view of the nurses interviewed it has not had any appreciable effect on the content of their work. The terminal in the duty room, which is quite unsuitable for dialogue with the Information System, demonstrates the limitations of the technology as a work tool for the nurses. Originally monitors had been installed with the micro-printers to facilitate dialogue via coded entries. However, during the first few years of use, the monitors were not thought necessary, and so when defects arose they were removed and not replaced.

The main reason which limits use of the system by nurses is that little of the stored information is viewed by the nurses as relevant to nursing. For example, the laboratory results are of more use to the doctor than to the nurse. Administrative tasks, because of their routine nature, would be most amenable to computerisation but this has not occurred. Forms are still filled in by hand, the only change being a relatively minor one - the use of self-adhesive labels for patient details.

However, several nurses reported that the pressure of work often leaves insufficient time for their administrative duties, and therefore their completion is a cause of stress. The Netherlands study reported a similar finding, administrative and organisational tasks tend to take lowest priority compared with tasks which relate directly to patient care. The pressure on the ward sister is particularly great since, because she is the principal contact with the doctor, she carries out many of these administrative tasks. Yet she is one of the most highly skilled members of the nursing staff whose time is 'wasted' in routine clerical work. For this reason time-saving is one of the main arguments in favour of computerisation. In fact an information leaflet on the technology issued to hospital employees concludes, "You should have more time for the work for which you have been trained i.e. the care of the patient".

In the view of ward managers and nurses, time savings have not occurred. In fact there has been a general increase in administrative work. This is in part a consequence of more diagnostic and therapeutic services being available and therefore requested. In addition, in the recent past, time-consuming clerical duties have been transferred from central services to ward management; for example, keeping accounts of overtime worked and time-off due to staff.

Against these additional administrative tasks the small time saved by use of the self-adhesive labels can be off-set. Yet further time saving which might have been made - for example, by standardising and condensing the 30 or more forms used - had not been achieved. The net effect is increased time spent on administrative tasks.

The effect on work organisation:

Any changes in work organisation cannot be attributed simply to new technology, but must be considered in the context of the reorganisation of the wards within a department. The computer system has not brought about any organisational changes on its own account. The internal division of labour on the wards and work planning in particular have remained unaffected. This is not surprising considering that the computerisation has not directly affected the work content of nursing or even the performance of administrative tasks.

Changes have occurred however, by the creation of the departmental secretary role. The primary effect has been a channelling of most communications between the ward and other departments. In the initial changes this led to some friction between nurses and secretaries, but these were sorted out as the work became routine. From the nurses point of view there were no serious difficulties breaking off direct contact with other departments since these communications were already extremely formal in content and, because of the size of the hospital, anonymous.

The need for special measures outside of office hours imposed limitations and also led to a pile-up of work for the following day. This has remained an unsolved organisational problem. With high volumes of work and staff shortages these problems have exacerbated the stress factors.

In contrast, while the office is open it takes some pressure off the ward staff. They do not need to concern themselves with administrative details during admission, and even after admission the secretary attends to patients' requirements insofar as they concern the notification of relatives, the family doctor, clergy or social worker. The office, being centrally placed, also prevents undirected visitors intruding in the ward unchecked. It shields and acts as a buffer for the ward so that interference in the nursing work is minimised.

These relieving features are probably chiefly responsible for the general acceptance of the intermediary. However, the continued need for form filling, and subsequent entry by the secretary, is regarded as duplication of effort. Staff see the need for some further reorganisation, though not the elimination of the departmental office. On the contrary, there is a repeated request for office hours to be extended.

Nurses' views of the system:

The nurses were not keen to use the computer terminals themselves, although none of the respondents showed any particular aversion to, or fear of, such work. This probably contributed to their positive views about the role of the departmental secretaries. In response to the question of whether they would like a more decentralised system with fully interactive terminals in the duty room of each ward, one replied, "Yes, provided that each ward then has at least one part-time ward secretary". This in part recognises the increased workload that might accompany delegation to wards, but also suggests no enthusiasm for direct entry. An alternative way of organising decentralisation might provide autonomous ward terminals, but compensate for any extra work with additional nursing hours.

In general the attitude of the nurses to information technology could be described as indifference. Lack of direct personal experience as a system user, and difficulty in assessing any positive effects of the technology on one's own work situation do not motivate or offer the enthusiasm to seek extensions to the existing system useful to oneself. Proposals made to the nurses by outside agencies are initially treated with scepticism.

An example of the indifference engendered in the nurses by their experience of the technology is provided by an experiment that was carried out in the ward on computerised collection of data on patients' medication. The objective was to be able to provide lists of the daily distribution of medicines, to provide medication reports for patients' files, and to provide reports of patients' medication profiles over several days. Data collection was delegated to the nursing staff, using the telephone terminal for input.

Data entry was very difficult because of the need to use numerical codes (patient's number, medication code, dosage). Few of these were memorised. The complexity resulted in many input errors, which had to be corrected by hand on the print-out and re-entered. Most seriously data had to be hand-written outside of the computer centre's operating hours and entered later.

These difficulties, plus the fact that the function dealt only with secondary nursing duties, meant additional work for the nurses and overall nurses were extremely dissatisfied. The problems could not be resolved satisfactorily and the nursing management decided that nursing staff would no longer co-operate with the experiment, and no further data was collected. It appears that, through an experiment of this kind, the hospital management unintentionally, but rather effectively, managed to engender negative (or at best indifferent) attitudes. The nurses' already high workload was increased with no compensating benefits. The experiment, to an outside researcher, appears to have had inherent faults almost guaranteed to encourage nursing staff to view computerisation negatively. There appears to have been little or no effort made to respond to the nurses' needs as users of the system.

The departmental secretaries' views:

Since the departmental secretaries jobs were created by the computerisation, it is not possible to assess the effects on tasks formerly done without the computer. Although the secretary is solely responsible for operating the terminal her work does not consist exclusively of VDU operation. Other tasks include servicing the terminals in the duty-room, installing patients' telephones and issuing accounts, operating the small conveyor system, handling enquiries from relatives, consultants etc. The amount of VDU work depends mainly on the number of new patients admitted, and generally is confined to morning use. Thus although the work station is poorly designed, the variety of work makes the poor design of secondary importance to the secretaries.

The mix of duties can however be stressful when a number of tasks are required at the same time, and there is no obvious way of co-ordinating them or assigning priorities. Thus there are similarities between the nature of the nurses' and the secretaries work. Both groups have to respond to high demand and unforseen changes in demand. This perhaps leads to mutual understanding of each other's position. The nurses' acceptance of the office function and the secretaries' role forms the basis of the job satisfaction of the secretaries interviewed. They are conscious of providing meaningful support to the work of the wards.

The impact on the patients:

It should be clear from the description of the information system, and its impact on the nurses' work, that there are few opportunities for the patient to be even aware of the system. During admission the patients are likely to be aware that their data is being entered at a terminal since it is usually used simultaneously. If, as many patients have, the patient has already had contact with the hospital, they can appreciate the advantage of having their details already available in the system. Patients' views are moulded by their experience of the ward environment generally and probably negligibly by any direct contact with the computer system. Nor is it likely that there will be an indirect effect, mediated by any changed relationship with the nurses, since the nurses themselves experience little direct impact, as previously described. Thus there is no evidence of any impact on the patients - positive or negative.

2.8.5 Overview of the study

The German study has examined the impact of a Hospital Information System (HIS) in two departments each with four (20 bed) wards. From the department's point of view, the main purpose of the system is to maintain communications with the various departments which provide a service to the wards - for example laboratory tests, domestic services etc. The organisation of the system is partly-centralised in that most communications are channelled through the departmental secretary (a specially created role), who does all the data entry. Each ward also has a terminal in the duty room attached to it. However this is mainly used as a 'telex' terminal for receiving results back from the laboratory.

The HIS has had little or no direct impact on the nurses work, because its functions are essentially administrative, and even these are ones that are mainly peripheral to the main nursing activities. The nurses do not use the departmental office terminal at all themselves. They are, overall, indifferent to the HIS, seeing at best only marginal benefit to themselves or their own work (e.g. self-adhesive labels), but nor are they troubled by it. An earlier experiment with a ward based system for collecting information on medication administered to patients and providing reports was unsuccessful and was withdrawn when the nursing management withdrew cooperation. Thus, on the basis of past experience with information technology, the nurses have little to feel optimistic about. But they are pleased to leave the data entry work to the secretaries, carrying on themselves providing the necessary information on handwritten forms. The departmental secretaries are seen as useful to the nurses in that they take away some of the burden of admission administration and also act as a buffer protecting the ward from outside disturbances such as uncontrolled visits from patients' relatives. The secretaries themselves derive job satisfaction from being useful to the nurses.

There is no apparent impact of the HIS, or the associated reorganisations of work, on the patients. The nurses see themselves under a lot of work pressure, but this is attributable to staff shortages and the increased workload produced by the carrying out of more diagnostic and therapeutic procedures which are becoming increasingly available.

The German report also assesses indications that the introduction of information technology is proceeding in association with major rationalisations of hospital work, which may eventually reach the nursing process itself. These issues are developed and discussed more fully in section 3.2.1 of this report. Similarly, the report raises some important questions concerning the advantages and disadvantages of developing hospital information systems within a centralised or decentralised framework. These issues are discussed further in section 3.2.2.

3.0   DISCUSSION AND CONCLUSIONS

The main aim of this report has been to describe and assess the impact of new technology on nursing staff and patients in hospitals. Five of the six case studies have examined the stressors that exist in the Intensive Care environment. It is here that nurses and patients come most directly into contact with new technology. As well as assessing the extent to which new technology alleviates or compounds the stress found in a modern hospital ward, the studies investigated the success with which nursing staff work with the technology and the problems that have arisen. The important question - to what extent does the technology undermine or distract from the traditional 'caring' skills of nurses? - has been addressed.

This report also assesses the wider impact of new technology on nursing. In particular it examines the use of information systems in 'ordinary' wards, and anticipates changes that may occur in the nursing process itself in the near future. Finally, based on the findings and conclusions, the report puts forward a set of recommendations on changes that need to take place in the way that new technology is being developed and implemented within the health services.

3.1   The Impact of Intensive Care Technologies

The conceptual framework put forward in the introduction indicates that the impact of new technology on patients in intensive care could be either direct or indirect. Patients could experience the direct consequences of being 'wired up' to a web of equipment, they might also experience indirect consequences through a changed relationship with the nurses. There may be a direct impact on nursing staff, the users of the technology. Alternatively, the impact may derive from a change in the organisation of the unit's work, introduced in tandem with the technological developments.

To test these possibilities, in this section, we draw together the evidence for the impact on intensive care units, and on the jobs of nursing staff. We also examine the nurses' and the patients' experiences of the technology.

3.1.1 Job characteristics, environmental supports and stressors

A number of characteristics of nursing work emerge as commonly occurring stressors for nursing staff. These are:

(1)   A high work pace and frequent overload. This stressor is particularly pervasive in intensive care units, especially during new admissions when a number of complex procedures must be carried out rapidly and efficiently. In some circumstances a patient must be 'decanted' to a follow-up ward to make room for the emergency. This is particularly onerous.

(2)   Rapid decision making and a high level of responsibility. In intensive care, patients depend for their survival on constant attention and relatively frequent interventions from nursing staff. This places greater responsibility on staff than in 'ordinary' wards where recovery to a greater extent is based on 'natural' (non-interventionist) healing processes. Moreover emergencies are relatively common in intensive care and, combined with the heavy workload, place considerable stress on nursing staff. This is particularly severe when a doctor is not immediately available and the nurses must make vital decisions - perhaps on whether to summon a doctor.

(3)   The work pressure is cumulative, and combines with the shiftwork, necessary to provide 24 hour cover, to induce fatigue. This is particularly severe when long shifts are worked (see the Irish study), or when there is a need for extensive overtime (see the Danish study).

(4)   Relating to seriously ill or dying patients and their relatives. This stress is a feature of all intensive care units, and is exacerbated by being involved in the application of therapeutic procedures which are intrusive and painful to patients.

(5)   Working with inexperienced staff. In several hospitals qualified nurses felt under greater pressure because they knew that their colleagues were not fully trained and therefore could not assume equal responsibility.

The following stress factors were identified as relating directly to the use of new technology:

(1)   Enhanced cognitive demands. Although monitoring technology may remove some of the burden of constant vigilance, the equipment is complex and frequently requires sophisticated interpretations.

(2)   Poor design and equipment failures. Several of the studies reported that the monitoring equipment produced frequent 'false alarms'. These were particularly stressful to nursing staff, especially when, as a result of poor design, it was difficult to decide immediately whether the alarm was in fact false.

(3)   Lack of adequate training. This was the most commonly reported problem and stressor - and perhaps the most serious. As a consequence of insufficient training in the use of the equipment (frequently no more than the supplier's introduction, or learning on the job from partially knowledgeable colleagues) the other problems were magnified. That is, the cognitive demands on staff were increased and false alarms made more difficult to diagnose.

(4)   Ethical questions. The technology makes it more possible to sustain life. Several nurses commented that this could raise difficult questions in their own minds. Although the doctors had the formal responsibility, the nurses were faced with the question of, in what circumstances, a patient's life should be sustained if it was likely to result in only partial recovery and a future 'low grade' life. Also, since the technology was sometimes a scarce resource, questions arose about priorities for its use when no equipment was immediately available for a patient who could benefit from it.

The problem of high workload is reported in all case studies. It serves to magnify the effects of many of the other stress factors. There appear to be a number of causes for this common finding:

(a)   There appears to be a general shortage of nursing staff in hospital units. The Netherlands report suggests that shortages do not just occur in high technology units. In fact they can be worse in low technology units because, in a situation of fixed overall health budgets, increased resources for high technology units have the effect of 'draining' resources from other units.

(b)   Advances in medicine and technology make possible more diagnostic and therapeutic procedures. These usually involve nurses in extra work, for example, carrying out the procedure or keeping administrative records of tests performed outside the unit. Since some of these procedures are invasive to patients, more time is required providing psychosocial support.

(c)   Over recent years a policy has been widely introduced that leads to patients spending less time in hospital, and less time in the intensive care unit. The consequence is that the same number (or more) administrative, diagnostic and therapeutic procedures have to be carried out during a shorter stay. This intensifies the nurses' work.

This catalogue of stressors is, to some extent at least, off-set by some positive job characteristics and environmental supports. These are:

(1)   High job quality. Nurses, particularly in intensive care, experience a high degree of meaningfulness, responsibility, independence, variety and scope for development in their work. The other side of the 'pressure' coin is a responsible job held in high esteem by society, and by patients who are usually very grateful.

(2)   Opportunities. Intensive care in particular provides opportunities for nurses to enhance their skills, and achieve promotion and increased pay.

(3)   Social supports. This factor can be either positive or negative, depending on the 'climate' in the unit or hospital. For example, the Danish study reports good relations within the unit between colleagues and with superiors. The atmosphere is seen as supportive and non-hierarchical. On the other hand the Irish study reports a bureaucratic climate and lack of recognition for nurses. 'Team work' is seen as poor and unsupportive. The Italian report comments that relations between nurses in the intensive care unit are good, but that the introduction of computer-based monitoring equipment has reduced the need - and opportunity - for communication between nurses, particularly at the point where one shift hands over to the next. Thus the study reports a lack of support amongst staff.

3.1.2 Stress and coping

The Danish, Italian and Netherlands studies have assessed nurses' stress reactions to their work environment. Overall, intensive care nurses do not appear to exhibit serious stress symptoms. The Danish report found indications of fatigue and psychological stress but few psychosomatic symptoms.

Nurses who exhibited more symptoms tended to be young, relatively inexperienced, and without prior work experience of new technology. The Italian report found stress levels in the intensive care unit a little higher than in the hyperbaric treatment centre, but not high compared with levels experienced by other groups of workers. However because of the shift system, fatigue did accumulate over several shifts, and was only relieved by the two day break. The Netherlands report found a slight tendency for nurses in the lower technology units to experience greater stress.

Thus the extensive environmental stressors result in relatively mild stress symptoms. This may, in part, be due to the compensating positive qualities of the nurses' job. It may also indicate that nurses who experience more stress transfer to a less demanding work environment. Some of the studies examined the ways that the nurses said they coped with stress. In the Irish study many nurses found it necessary to 'unwind' in their own time after work. They experienced little opportunity to influence their working environment which they reported as bureaucratic and unsupportive. The Danish study found that the nurses experiencing most stress also tended to resort to individual coping strategies. It may be that the more experienced nurses felt more able to influence the sources of stress since the environment was seen as generally supportive. This appears to be the more effective strategy for dealing with stressors if circumstances permit it. However, all studies reported the time pressure that nurses work under. The Netherlands report points out that, under such circumstances, there is not enough time or opportunity to participate in planning or other decisions which might make it possible to influence the work environment.

3.1.3 Using new technology

The majority of nurses see the benefits of using new technology, and in particular its life sustaining potential. However, they also experience serious problems with its use, which fall into two broad categories – problems with design and reliability, and problems resulting from inadequate training. False alarms from monitoring equipment are a major source of anxiety and are focused on by the Danish, Italian and UK reports. Insufficient training is featured in all the reports.

In the introduction five hypotheses were presented. These were qualitative changes typical of the effect of introducing new technology into jobs characterised by high skill levels, such as found in nursing. The hypotheses are now reviewed in the light of the evidence available from the case studies in intensive care units:

(1)   There is a shift from manual to intellectual skills. This seems to be the case, particularly for computer-based monitoring technologies. There is less need for movement of nurses around the ward if monitoring is done from a central point. The equipment can be complex to operate and usually produces extensive print-outs which need sophisticated interpretation.

(2)   There is an increased distance between the users (nurses) and the product (the patients). Most of the intensive care case studies have confirmed this hypothesis - at least for some nurses. There appears to be variation in the extent to which nurses compensate for this distancing effect. In some environments there appears to be little opportunity, in others the nurses try to provide additional direct support to alleviate some of the anxiety induced by invasive treatments.

(3)   There is a shift from concrete visible targets to more abstract ones. Monitoring technologies rely on quantified measures of vital functions. These are the basis on which alarms operate and they become the basis on which nurses judge a patient's state of health. There is less direct assessment of how the patient appears.

(4)   Regulation and intervention in the work process (patient care) is based on a model of the work process which is not necessarily accessible or directly observable to the user (the nurse). This hypothesis is not confirmed by the evidence from the case studies. Although technology monitors vital functions there is no evidence that it regulates treatment without human intervention. Alarms are always a signal to the nurses that intervention may be necessary, and it is they who must make a decision. The unreliability of the equipment makes it unlikely that nurses will become deskilled by its use or fully dependent on its functioning.

(5)   There is a need for increased skills which must be regularly updated. This is certainly the case. A major problem arises because the necessary facilities are not generally available in most hospitals.

3.1.4 Patients' responses to new technology

The Danish, Irish and Italian studies interviewed patients who had direct experience of intensive care. Generally patients had very positive views of the service they had received and were particularly grateful to the nurses. There did not appear to be any evidence that patients felt 'distanced' from nursing staff as a result of the technology.

However the Irish, Italian and Netherlands studies report that the technology and the physical environment can be intrusive and invoke anxiety. The Italian study reports that patients' relatives would have liked more information about the equipment in use. Invasive procedures also reduce patient mobility and bring a greater risk of infection. The UK study points out that the policy of shortest possible stay in a unit can create a 'conveyor-belt' environment.

The environment can be stressful for patients, and this seems to depend on what support is provided by nursing staff to compensate, and on the environment itself. In some units, several patients were in a single ward and therefore shared the same environment. The Italian report highlights a phenomena referred to as 'Intensive Care Syndrome' in which patients experience temporal-spatial disorientation and almost total amnesia of the period in the unit. This may be attributed to a 'sensory deprivation effect', induced by no windows and constant lighting, and lack of routines and other cues to differentiate day and night in the unit. It may also be a mechanism which patients use to 'switch off' from the distress of other patients being experienced around them. Their own invasive treatment may also be a cause, and the study found a tendancy for patients to tear off monitoring or treatment equipment. Since this endangers the patient's life, doctors administer a massive sedation. This may be a cause of amnesia.

Individual rooms may provide a more positive environment, adaptable to the needs of the individual patient. However there may be negative consequences for the nurses, who derive support from being with their colleagues and simultaneously being able to observe patients from a central point. Remote computer-based monitoring allows the nurses to monitor from a central point even when the patients are in single rooms, but makes it difficult to directly observe the patients. However it may contribute to the positive team work within the unit.

3.1.5 'Caring' and 'curing' aspects of nursing

'Caring' is the traditional autonomous nursing role to complement the 'curing' work of doctors. In modern hospitals it includes the basic physical care and psychosocial care that all patients need. 'Curing' on the other hand emphasises technical procedures, usually carried out for diagnostic or treatment purposes. Most curing activities are under the responsibility of doctors. The boundary between what doctors do and what nurses do is not well defined. It varies from unit to unit and, to some extent, depends on the availability of doctors, especially in acute situations. The Netherlands study has assessed the caring and curing components of the tasks performed by nurses. All tasks can be placed on a two-dimensional chart indicating the proportion of caring and curing that they entail, as judged by the nurses themselves according to a definition supplied by the researchers.

In the introduction the question was posed, has the balance between caring and curing changed as a result of using new technology? The evidence from the Netherlands study clearly indicates that many more curing activities take place in high technology units than in low technology ones. Correspondingly, low technology nurses carry out more caring activities. This appears to be a direct consequence of the vastly increased number of technical procedures entailed in the use of equipment in intensive care. It is also a consequence of patients spending less time in the hospital. In both types of unit nurses would prefer to spend more time on psychosocial care. The study identifies a 'hierarchy' of activities carried out by nurses:

(1)   Technical nursing.
(2)   Basic physical care and domestic duties.

(3)   Psychosocial care.

(4)   Organisational activities.

Thus technical procedures take top priority, and when under pressure there is insufficient time for psychosocial care or organisational activities. This latter category includes time spent planning the unit's activities and participating in decision making. The other case studies, although not adopting such quantitative techniques as the Netherlands study, support this general conclusion. Caring (and organising) activities get squeezed due to the priority of technical procedures combined with a shortage of available time. The extent of this 'squeezing out' seems to depend mainly on how much work pressure the nurses are under.

3.2   The Impact of New Technology on Nurses and Patients

The previous section has examined the impact of intensive care technologies. This section broadens the focus, brings in the findings of the German study on the use of information systems, and assesses the way that the nursing process is changing and may change further in the future.

3.2.1   The rationalisation of nursing work

The case studies of intensive care nursing have revealed that nursing is becoming more technical and based on specific procedures for the diagnosis and treatment of patients. The Netherlands study has found evidence that intensive care nurses have less autonomy in their work because of the need to make interventions on pre-determined criteria and to follow pre-determined procedures. It is also argued that because high technology health care consumes extra resources (it is both more capital and more labour intensive), and because it is being developed in a context of predominantly fixed budgets, the result is a net 'draining' of resources from low technology units.

The Netherlands report also identified a trend towards independent functions which, the report anticipates, will result in the nursing profession, in its classic form, ceasing to exist. New professions will be created, and patient care will be provided by separate professions for:

(1) Physical care and domestic work: tasks requiring minimal training in patient care.

(2) Psychosocial care: tasks involving psychologists, social workers, sick visitors etc.

(3) Curing activities: tasks performed by paramedical workers trained in technical procedures.

(4) Medical advice: decisions made by medical consultants.

Were this degree of fragmentation and specialisation to take place, a likely consequence would be isolation of workers within each branch of health care and greater problems of co-ordination. Nursing provides a valuable contribution which would be lost if the above trends continue extensively. This is the opportunity and ability to provide integrated support to patients, to respond to their physical and emotional needs, by providing information, care, guidance and organisation.

However, even in intensive care, and especially in ordinary wards, nursing cannot as yet be described as a formalised process. It is still based, to a considerable extent, on intuition and personal judgement. There tends not to be a high degree of formalisation in nursing management and the keeping of records which would be used to assess nursing performance. In other words, the nursing process has not been 'rationalised' in a way that would make it readily amenable to computerisation. This would require the availability of formal techniques and measuring instruments (records etc.) to analyse and classify the nursing process.

One reason for non-rationalisation may be that, because of the constant time pressures on the wards, there is not sufficient opportunity to devote the time to the organising of activities that would be required. Another reason for the relative failure to apply information technology to the nursing process may be economic. Since one aim of such developments would be to safeguard or improve the quality of health care, and to professionalise further the nursing service, it may also require additional resources and therefore expenditure. There are likely to be additional capital costs and no reduction in labour costs for <u>process</u> technologies that aid the nursing process itself. Any time saving innovations would be fully offset by the creation of new activities.

The German study provides indications that the same may also apply to the introduction of <u>information systems</u> technology. The study examined the impact of a Hospital Information System which was used by wards for communicating with centrally provided services (laboratories, domestic services, etc.). Communications with the network were made through the specially created role of departmental secretary. Nursing staff did not use the system directly themselves and continued to record information on manual forms which were passed on to the secretary.

Nevertheless nurses have positive expectations of future uses of information technology. They hope it will reduce the amount of administration and paperwork they need to do, by rationalising the current system. However in the current climate, any time savings that did arise might not directly benefit the nurses by reducing their workload, but might lead to a reduction in staffing levels.

3.2.2 The consequences of centralised and decentralised systems

If nurses are asked to supply data for a central network (perhaps for audit or accounting purposes) they are unlikely to do so with any enthusiasm or consistency unless they perceive some benefits to the nursing process or to themselves. Yet many hospital information systems collect information while remaining peripheral to the nursing process. The German report describes an experiment with a computer system which failed because it required nurses to provide information that would be used for medication assessment. It failed because the system was difficult for the nurses to use and gave them no direct benefit. The nursing management withdrew cooperation from the project when the problems could not be resolved satisfactorily.

The main system described in the German report, which is partially centralised, also provides no direct benefit to the nurses. But it is tolerated because the data entry is done by secretaries, who in addition help the nurses by acting as a buffer between the wards and the outside world - in particular relatives of patients. The German report also describes a decentralised system in another German hospital. This requires nurses to make direct entries during their nursing activities. But it fails because in practice there is not sufficient time to make entries during a busy ward round, and the benefit to nurses - a print-out of an order form and protocol - is only available from a printer located several flights of stairs away! The report also outlines a decentralised system in an American hospital (Cook, 1982), which does succeed in relieving the nurses' clerical workload. It uses direct entry by <u>doctors</u> during their normal work. The system is of benefit to nursing staff and makes them into 'information users' rather than 'information suppliers'.

There appears to have been too little consideration of the nurses' role as professional workers in the design of hospital information systems. If computer applications are to <u>benefit</u> the nursing process and assist nurses, either by reducing the workload or providing useful information, they are going to need the participation of nurses in their development.

3.3   The Involvement of Nurses in the Development of New Technology

A recurring theme in the case studies is the lack of involvement that nursing staff have had in the introduction of new technology, even though they were its main users. It is common for new equipment to 'arrive' for almost immediate use. Sometimes nurses are involved at a fairly advanced stage of installation when most of the technical and organisational decisions have been made, and the technology must be 'adapted' to the local environment and work situation.

Many of the nurses commented that they felt the technology could be of greater benefit to patient care, and less stressful to them, if they were more involved in its development, and the plans for its use. However there appear to be at least four major pre-conditions for effective participation to take place:

(1)   There must be a willingness on the part of hospital management for such involvement to take place. This might result from a recognition that more <u>effective</u> use of the technology could be a consequence.

(2)   Nursing staff must <u>want</u> to participate in planning the developments in their work. The evidence suggests that they do, but

(3)   The high workload results in insufficient time and opportunity to get involved in organisational activities. Therefore more time needs to be made available.

(4)   To make a useful contribution to technical developments nurses need sufficient practical experience of the potential and likely consequences of using new technology. This requires concrete training and practice <u>prior</u> to the installation of equipment.

4.0   RECOMMENDATIONS

An important aim of the research has been to present findings of practical relevance, which may be used to improve the work experiences of hospital staff, and the service as experienced by patients. To this end a set of recommendations are now offered on the way new technology should be developed and implemented within the health services. These recommendations result directly from the findings reported in each of the six national case studies, and from the conclusions of those studies. In this, the consolidated report, they are presented in seven broad categories.

These recommendations have been fed-back to the researchers who undertook the six national studies. The recommendations have received their support and approval. In situations where amplifying comments have been made by the researchers, these views have been incorporated. Thus, although the case studies have employed a wide range of methods in a variety of environments, the recommendations reported here represent a consensus view that emerges directly from the research.

(1)   More and better training

The introduction of new technology requires that adequate training be provided to nursing staff. Current training, which tends to be provided by equipment suppliers and supplemented by learning from experience, is not sufficient. Training should be seen as the hospital's responsibility, and sufficient time and resources should be made available for it. It should not be isolated 'technology-training' but be seen as an instrument of better nursing. Training should include instruction in functional principles, sources of common malfunction and how to rectify faults, how to distinguish true and false alarms. It should be available to all staff in the unit so that nurses do not become dependent on one or two 'experts' who may not be directly available in an emergency. It may also be necessary to provide simple equipment handbooks designed specifically for the workplace and equipment in question. Nurses should also receive advice and support on how to integrate the technology into their daily work so as to maintain good contact with patients. Associated with on-going training in the use of new technology it may be desirable to provide courses which perhaps use role-playing techniques in, for example, the counselling of dying patients.

(2)   User-centred design

The technology should be 'user-centred' and support the needs of the nursing process (rather than be merely superficially appealing). In the case of Hospital Information Systems, nurses should be 'information users' and not just 'information providers'. Moreover, data collection and entry should not interfere with the nursing process itself, and where possible direct input of information by doctors should be encouraged. Since frequent interruptions occur in nursing work the system should allow breaking-off from an activity and then its resumption at the same point at a later occasion. It is important that monitoring technology is designed to good 'human factors' principles to avoid the stressful problems of a high level of false-alarms.

(3)   Support for nursing staff

The introduction of new technology increases the need for ensuring that mechanisms exist to provide support to nurses in their work. A non-bureaucratic, supportive environment, with 'team work' between nurses and doctors, reduces stress for nurses. Consideration should be given to whether there are adequate opportunities for nurses to communicate with each other, especially when handing over to the next shift. To improve communication and support amongst nursing staff group discussions should be organised on the organisation of patient care, communication with doctors, dealing with relatives, work organisation, and use of equipment, etc.

(4)   Ensuring care of patients

There is evidence that patients suffer if placed in an alienating environment without sufficient personal support. For example, they may develop 'intensive care syndrome'. The environment should be designed to allow 'normal' sleeping and waking patterns wherever possible. It is important that patients have sufficient privacy. This will require partitions in large wards or a move towards smaller rooms. It is important that patients do not overhear doctors and nurses talking about the state of other patients. Since new technology, and other developments, are leading to relatively more 'curing' activities, there should be a conscious and deliberate increase in time available for 'caring' activities. This should enable more psychosocial support from nursing staff, including explanations about the purposes and uses of high technology equipment.

(5) Integration of tasks, jobs and units

The development and use of new technology is leading to increased specialisation in nursing work. Nurses in high technology units report too many technical procedures, nurses in low technology units report not enough. At the level of the tasks (curing and caring), the job (technical nursing, domestic duties, social work, administration), and the unit (high technology, low technology) there is a need for re-integration to stem and reverse the trend towards over specialisation. This should result in an improvement in the quality of nursing work and in patient care.

(6) Participation in decision making

Generally nurses have had little active involvement in the changes taking place on their wards. Mechanisms need to be set up to allow and ensure more involvement in ward organisation, planning and policy making. In particular, nursing staff should be actively involved in systems development and implementation. To be effective this requires practical experience on the part of nurses, so 'model experiments' should be set up as pilots to new developments. These must be systematically evaluated for their consequences for the quality of patient care and nursing work.

(7) Increased staffing levels

One of the most commonly reported stressors in nursing work is 'work overload'. This is both at acute periods, associated with admissions, and also a cumulative fatigue effect. The overload exists in high and low technology units because of the 'draining' strategy. There is a particular shortage of suitably experienced staff. Moreover, many of the other recommendations, if they are to be implemented effectively, will require the nurses to have sufficient time available. It is clear that an effect of using new technology is not to reduce the nurses' workload, in fact the reverse. It therefore comes as an unavoidable conclusion that the most important direct improvement in patient care and the quality of nursing work would be made if staffing levels were increased. The increased nursing time should be used to implement the other recommendations.

5.0   REFERENCES

Agervold, M. and Kristensen, O.S. (1985). The Impact of New Technology on Experienced Workers. European Foundation for the Improvement of Living and Working Conditions, Dublin.

Bernhard, P. (1983). Psychological aids for the personnel of intensive care units. In Hannick, Wendt and Lawin (eds.), Psychosomatics of Intensive Medicine. Stuttgart, New York.

Bishop, V. (1983). Stress in intensive care unit. Occupational Health, 35 (12), 537-543.

Broadbent, D. et al. (1982). The cognitive failures questionnaire and its correlates. British Journal of Clinical Psychology, 21, 1-16.

Caplan, R.D. et al. (1975). Job Demands and Work Health: Main Effects and Occupational Differences. US Government Printing Office, Washington DC.

Claus, K., Bailey, J. and Selye, H. (1980). Living with Stress and Promoting Well-Being. The CU Mosby Company, London, Toronto.

Cook, M. (1982). Using computers to enhance professional practice. Nursing Times, September 15, 1542-1544.

Cruickshank, P.J. (1982). Patient stress and the computer in the consulting room. Social Science Medicine, 16 (14), 1371-1376.

Cruickshank, P.J. (1984). Computers in medicine: Patients' attitudes. Journal of the Royal College of General Practitioners, 34, 77-80.

Dohrenwend, B.S. and Dohrenwend, B.P. (eds.) (1974). Stressful Life Events: Their Nature and Effects. John Wiley, New York.

Eden, D. (1982). Critical job events, acute stress and strain. Organisational Behaviour and Human Performance, 30, 312-329.

Farmer, E.S. (1977). The effects of the impact of technology on nursing. Glasgow West of Scotland Health Boards, Glasgow.

Farmer, E.S. (1978). The impact of technology on nursing. Nursing Mirror, September 28, 17-20.

Faulkner, W. and Arnold, E. (eds.) (1985). Smothered by Invention: Technology in Women's lives. Pluto Press, London.

Gay, E.G. et al. (1971). Manual for the Minnesota importance questionnaire. Bulletin 54, Minnesota Studies in Vocational Rehabilitation, University of Minnesota.

Goldberg, D.P. and Hillier, V.F. (1979). A scaled version of the general health questionnaire. Psychological Medicine, 9, 139-145.

Gray-Toft, P. and Anderson, J.C. (1981). Stress among hospital nursing staff: Its causes and effects. Social Science Medicine, 15, 639-647.

Hackman, J.R. and Oldham, G.R. (1975). Development of the Job Diagnostic survey. Journal of Applied Psychology, 60, 159-170.

Hannich, H.J., Wendt, M. and Lawin, P. (eds.) (1983). Psychosomatics of intensive medicine. Stuttgart, New York.

Hepworth, S. and Fitter, M.J. (1981). Nurses' attitudes to computers in hospitals. Memo No. 419, MRC/ESRC Social and applied Psychology Unit, University of Sheffield.

Huckaby, L.M.D. and Jagla, B. (1979). Nurse's stress factors in the intensive care unit. Journal of Nursing Administration, 9 (2), 21.

Jacobsen, S.F. (1978). Nurses' stress in intensive and non-intensive care units. In S.F. Jacobson and H.M. McGrath (eds.), Nurses Under Stress. John Wiley & Sons, New York.

Jokinen, M. and Poyhonen, T. (1980). Stress and Other Occupational Health Problems Afflicting Practical Nurses. Institute of Occupational Health, Helsinki.

Jones, J. et al. (1979). What the patients say: A study of reactions to an ICU. Intensive Care Medicine, 5 (2), 89-92.

Karasek, R.A. (1979). Job demands, job decision latitude and mental strain: Implications for job redesign. Administrative Science Quarterly, 24, 285-308.

Kornfeld, D.S. (1969). Psychiatric view of the ICU. British Medical Journal, 1, 108.

Lazarus, R.S., Cohen, J.B. and Folman, S. (1980). Psychological stress and adaptation - Some unresolved issues. In M. Selye (ed.), Guide to Stress Research. Von Nostrand, New York.

McCarthy, E. (1979). Women's roles and organisational context: A study of interactive effects. Unpublished dissertation, Department of Psychology, University College, Dublin.

Moos, R. (1981). Work Environment Scale Manual. Consulting Psychologists Press, Palto Alto, California.

Parkes, K.R. (1982). Occupational stress among student nurses: A natural experiment. Journal of Applied Psychology, 67 (6), 784-796.

Potter, A.R. (1981). Computers in general practice: The patient's voice. Journal of the Royal College of General Practitioners, 31, 83-85.

Pringle, M., Robins, S. and Brown, G. (1984). The Patient's view. British Medical Journal, 288, 28 January.

Redfern, S.J. (1979). The charge nurse: Job attitudes and occupational stability. PhD thesis, University of Aston, Birmingham.

Reichle, M.J. (1975). Psychological stress in the intensive care unit. Nurses Digest, 3, 12-15.

Reznikoff, M. et al. (1967). Attitudes towards computers among employees of a psychiatric hospital. Mental Hygiene, 51, 419-425.

Rosenberg, M. et al. (1967). Attitudes of nursing students towards computers. Nursing Outlook, 15, 44-46.

Quinn, R.P. and Staines, G.L. (1979). The 1977 Quality of Employment Survey. Institute for Social Research, University of Michigan.

Selye, H. (1976) The Stress of Life. McGraw Hill, New York.

Spielberger, C.D., Gorsuch, R., Lushene, R.E. (1970). STAI Manual - The State-Trait Anxiety Inventory. Consulting Psychologists Press, Palo Alto, California.

Startsman, T.S. and Robinson, R.E. (1972). The attitudes of medical and paramedical personnel towards computers. Computers and Biomedical Research, 5, 218-227.

Tabor, M. (1982). Health care job stresses. Occupational Health and Safety, 51 (12), 20-25.

Vredenberg, D.J. and Trinkous, R.J. (1983). An analysis of role stress among nurses. Journal of Vol Behaviour, 22 (1), 82-95.

Yates, L.J. (1983). Technology in nursing. Nurses Focus, 5 (2), 8.

Zielstorff, R.D. and Birckhead, L.M. (1978). Automation in nursing. Nursing Administration, March, 49-53.

The Impact of New Technology on Workers and Patients in the Health Services

Luxembourg: Office for Official Publications of the European Communities

87 - 116 pp. - 240 x 173 cm

EN

ISBN: 92-825-6797-4

Catalogue number: SY-48-87-363-EN-C

Price (excluding VAT) in Luxembourg:

ECU 10.60   BFR 450   UKL 8.00   USD 12.20   IRL 8.30

Venta y suscripciones · Salg og abonnement · Verkauf und Abonnement · Πωλήσεις και συνδρομές
Sales and subscriptions · Vente et abonnements · Vendita e abbonamenti
Verkoop en abonnementen · Venda e assinaturas

BELGIQUE/BELGIË

Moniteur belge/Belgisch Staatsblad
Rue de Louvain 40-42/Leuvensestraat 40-42
1000 Bruxelles/1000 Brussel
Tél. 512 00 26
CCP/Postrekening 000-2005502-27

Sous-dépôts/Agentschappen:
Librairie européenne/
Europese Boekhandel
Rue de la Loi 244/Wetstraat 244
1040 Bruxelles/1040 Brussel

CREDOC
Rue de la Montagne 34/Bergstraat 34
Bte 11/Bus 11
1000 Bruxelles/1000 Brussel

DANMARK

Schultz EF-publikationer
Møntergade 19
1116 København K
Tlf: (01) 14 11 95
Telecopier: (01) 32 75 11

BR DEUTSCHLAND

Bundesanzeiger Verlag
Breite Straße
Postfach 10 80 06
5000 Köln 1
Tel. (02 21) 20 29-0
Fernschreiber: ANZEIGER BONN 8 882 595
Telecopierer: 20 29 278

GREECE

G.C. Eleftheroudakis SA
International Bookstore
4 Nikis Street
105 63 Athens
Tel. 322 22 55
Telex 219410 ELEF

Sub-agent for Northern Greece:
Molho's Bookstore
The Business Bookshop
10 Tsimiski Street
Thessaloniki
Tel. 275 271
Telex 412885 LIMO

ESPAÑA

Boletín Oficial del Estado
Trafalgar 27
28010 Madrid
Tel. (91) 446 60 00

Mundi-Prensa Libros, S.A.
Castelló 37
28001 Madrid
Tel. (91) 431 33 99 (Libros)
          431 32 22 (Suscripciones)
          435 36 37 (Dirección)
Télex 49370-MPLI-E

FRANCE

Journal officiel
Service des publications
des Communautés européennes
26, rue Desaix
75727 Paris Cedex 15
Tél. (1) 45 78 61 39

IRELAND

Government Publications Sales Office
Sun Alliance House
Molesworth Street
Dublin 2
Tel. 71 03 09

or by post

Government Stationery Office
Publications Section
6th floor
Bishop Street
Dublin 8
Tel. 78 16 66

ITALIA

Licosa Spa
Via Lamarmora, 45
Casella postale 552
50 121 Firenze
Tel. 57 97 51
Telex 570466 LICOSA I
CCP 343 509

Subagenti:
Libreria scientifica Lucio de Biasio - AEIOU
Via Meravigli, 16
20 123 Milano
Tel. 80 76 79

Libreria Tassi
Via A. Farnese, 28
00 192 Roma
Tel. 31 05 90

Libreria giuridica
Via 12 Ottobre, 172/R
16 121 Genova
Tel. 59 56 93

GRAND-DUCHÉ DE LUXEMBOURG
et autres pays/and other countries

Office des publications officielles
des Communautés européennes
2, rue Mercier
L-2985 Luxembourg
Tél. 49 92 81
Télex PUBOF LU 1324 b
CCP 19190-81
CC bancaire BIL 8-109/6003/200

Abonnements/Subscriptions

Messageries Paul Kraus
11, rue Christophe Plantin
L-2339 Luxembourg
Tél. 49 98 888
Télex 2515
CCP 49242-63

NEDERLAND

Staatsdrukkerij- en uitgeverijbedrijf
Christoffel Plantijnstraat
Postbus 20014
2500 EA 's-Gravenhage
Tel. (070) 78 98 80 (bestellingen)

PORTUGAL

Imprensa Nacional
Casa da Moeda, E. P.
Rua D. Francisco Manuel de Melo, 5
1092 Lisboa Codex
Tel. 69 34 14
Telex 15328 INCM

Distribuidora Livros Bertrand Lda.
Grupo Bertrand, SARL
Rua das Terras dos Vales, 4-A
Apart. 37
2700 Amadora CODEX
Tel. 493 90 50 - 494 87 88
Telex 15798 BERDIS

UNITED KINGDOM

HM Stationery Office
HMSO Publications Centre
51 Nine Elms Lane
London SW8 5DR
Tel. (01) 211 56 56

Sub-agent:
Alan Armstrong & Associates Ltd
72 Park Road
London NW1 4SH
Tel. (01) 723 39 02
Telex 297635 AAALTD G

UNITED STATES OF AMERICA

European Community Information
Service
2100 M Street, NW
Suite 707
Washington, DC 20037
Tel. (202) 862 9500

CANADA

Renouf Publishing Co., Ltd
61 Sparks Street
Ottawa
Ontario K1P 5R1
Tel. Toll Free 1 (800) 267 4164
Ottawa Region (613) 238 8985-6
Telex 053-4936

JAPAN

Kinokuniya Company Ltd
17-7 Shinjuku 3-Chome
Shiniuku-ku
Tokyo 160-91
Tel. (03) 354 0131

Journal Department
PO Box 55 Chitose
Tokyo 156
Tel. (03) 439 0124